高等院校药学类专业双语实验教材

药用植物学双语实验

主　编　王建安　许崇梅

副主编　付英杰　李艳芝　唐金宝

编　委（以姓氏笔画为序）

王建安（济宁医学院）

付英杰（济宁医学院）

吕艳娜（潍坊医学院）

曲畅游（山东药品食品职业学院）

许崇梅（潍坊医学院）

李艳芝（济宁医学院）

高丽娜（济宁医学院）

唐金宝（潍坊医学院）

赛春梅（济宁医学院）

中国健康传媒集团

中国医药科技出版社

内 容 提 要

　　本教材是"高等院校药学类专业双语实验教材"中的一本。本套教材由济宁医学院联合潍坊医学院共同编写。为适应医药行业国际化对药学类人才的需求，结合目前大学生英语水平普遍较高的特点，本套教材采用英汉双语编写。本教材由两部分组成。第一部分介绍了药用植物学实验基本技术。第二部分药用植物学实验部分是本书的主要内容，共 17 个实验。

　　本教材适合高等药学院校药学类专业使用。

图书在版编目（CIP）数据

药用植物学双语实验 / 王建安，许崇梅主编. —北京：中国医药科技出版社，2019.2
高等院校药学类专业双语实验教材
ISBN 978-7-5214-0729-7

Ⅰ．①药… Ⅱ．①王… Ⅲ．①药用植物学–实验–双语教学–高等学校–教材 Ⅳ．①Q949.95-33

中国版本图书馆 CIP 数据核字（2019）第 010249 号

美术编辑　　陈君杞
版式设计　　易维鑫

出版　**中国健康传媒集团** ｜ 中国医药科技出版社
地址　北京市海淀区文慧园北路甲 22 号
邮编　100082
电话　发行：010-62227427　邮购：010-62236938
网址　www.cmstp.com
规格　787×1092mm　¹⁄₁₆
印张　6
字数　139 千字
版次　2019 年 2 月第 1 版
印次　2019 年 2 月第 1 次印刷
印刷　三河市双峰印刷装订有限公司
经销　全国各地新华书店
书号　ISBN 978-7-5214-0729-7
定价　**16.00 元**

版权所有　盗版必究
举报电话：010-62228771
本社图书如存在印装质量问题请与本社联系调换

目 录

第一部分 药用植物学实验基本技术

第一节 显微镜的构造与使用

一、显微镜的构造

显微镜的种类不尽相同，有的简单，有的复杂，而且各有专门用途。本实验课所用的是最常见的复式显微镜。它们的基本结构相同，都是由光学部分和机械部分组成（图1-1）。

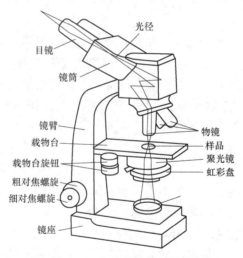

图1-1 复式显微镜的结构

光学部分：物镜、目镜、镜筒、聚光器和反光镜。

机械部分：转换器、粗准焦螺旋、细准焦螺旋、镜臂、载物台（镜台，上面装有压片夹或移动标本制片的推进器）、镜柱、倾斜关节、镜座。

显然，以上显微镜的结构和在中学期间用过的基本相同，也就是说中学时所用的显微镜也是一种复式显微镜。两者最大不同就是调节进入镜筒光线的装置不同，即中学所用的显微镜是转动遮光器以变更遮光器的光圈，而我们现在使用的显微镜其光线调节是由聚光器及附属结构来实现的。聚光器位于载物台的孔下方，由两块或数块透镜组成。它的作用是聚集反射镜反射来的光线，并将其射入镜筒，以增强标本的亮度。聚光器可通过聚光器升降螺旋的转动进行上、下调节以求适宜光度：向下降落亮度减少，向上提升则亮度加强。

1

如果显微镜视野内可见到窗框的投影，除改变反射镜方向外，也可将聚光器适当下调。聚光器的下面附有虹彩光圈，也可称光栏，由十几片金属片组成，推动其把手可用来控制聚光器口径的大小和照射面，以调节光的强弱。光强时缩小光圈，光弱时放大光圈。虹彩光圈下面还附设一金属圆圈，根据需要可放置某种色调的滤光片，以提高观察效果和突出某一部位成像的效果，这多在照相时使用。

二、显微镜的使用

1. 取用、放回等搬动显微镜时，必须一手握持镜臂，一手托住镜座，使镜身直立，不可用一只手倾斜提携，以免摔落目镜、反射镜以及镜座。

2. 要轻拿轻放。将显微镜置于实验台上时，镜臂朝向自己，略偏向左方距实验桌的边缘约 30 mm 处，右侧可放记录本或绘图纸等。

3. 使用显微镜前，首先要调节好光线，在实验室可以利用灯光或自然光，但不能用直射的阳光，以免损伤眼睛。首先转动转换器，使目镜、低倍物镜（通常是 10× 物镜）和通光孔成一直线，然后转动粗准焦螺旋，使物镜与载物台相距 7～8 mm，接着先把聚光器提上，打开可变光栏，在用左眼观察目镜中视野的同时，转动反光镜，使视野的光线最明亮、最均匀。如果靠近光源或光源较强，可用平面的反光镜；如果光源距离较远或光源较弱，可用凹面的反光镜。

4. 把要观察的切片置于载物台上，用推进器或手移动载玻片，使标本正对通光孔的中央（若无推进器的，移动后应用压片夹固定）。接着用左眼观察，若没看见标本，可慢慢旋转粗准焦螺旋，使镜筒慢慢上升，直到能看清标本为止。此时若物像不在视野中央，可移动载玻片，使标本物像出现在视野中央。移动时就记住显微镜中形成的物像是放大的倒像，故改变图像在视野中的位置时，需要朝相反的方向移动，或叫"对着干"，即偏右了向右移动玻片；反之亦然。然后再用细准焦螺旋进行调节（注意：细准焦螺旋是显微镜上机械部件中最易损坏的部件，要尽量保护。通常使用低倍物镜观察时，用粗准焦螺旋调焦就可以得到满意的效果，在此情况下，尽量不用或少用细准焦螺旋。使用高倍物镜如需要用细准焦螺旋调焦时，转动量也最好不要大于半圈）。

5. 进行观察时，一定要双眼睁开，做到左眼观察，右眼看绘图，同时要先从低倍镜下观察起。先了解制片时切片的情况，如需详细观察制片中某一部分的细微结构，则先在低倍下找到合适的位置，并移到中央，然后转动镜头转换器，用较高倍的物镜观察。如尚需要用更高倍的物镜进一步观察某一部分的结构，则可重复以上步骤。在观察过程中，由于材料、目镜、物镜放大倍数等不同，所需光线强弱也不同，则靠调节聚光器上、下位置和光栏光圈大小来实现。

6. 本实验通常使用高倍物镜，基本上能达到目的。如观察材料欲放大 1000 倍以上时，则需使用油浸物镜（即 100×）。使用油镜时，采用的目镜跟使用其他倍数的物镜时一样，可用 10×，15×，25× 等。观察时必须先用高倍物镜找到要观察的部位，调至视野中央后，再转动粗准焦螺旋。提高镜筒，转动镜头转换器，使油镜头与镜筒相对，然后在所要观察材料的盖玻片上面，在正对通光孔的中央部位加一滴直径约半厘米的石蜡油或柏木油。随后从显微镜侧面观察，操纵粗准焦螺旋，使镜筒下降至油镜头浸入油内，并正好与盖玻片相融，然后用左眼靠近目镜，细心观察视野，旋转粗准焦螺旋，使镜筒缓慢地向上提升，当刚刚看出不甚清楚的物像时，就换用细准焦螺旋，再进行调节，调至物像清晰为止。

观察完毕，提起镜筒，当即用擦镜纸擦去镜头上的石蜡油。若用柏木油（也称香柏油），需用擦镜纸先擦去镜头的柏木油，再用擦镜纸蘸少许二甲苯轻轻擦之，最后用干净的擦镜纸擦净。标本制片上的石蜡油（或柏木油）用同法擦去。

7. 每一种标本观察完毕后，必须在低倍镜下取出，若在高倍镜下或油镜下观察也必须转换至低倍镜下（或将镜筒提起一定高度）方可取出。这样可避免损坏玻片标本和镜头。若在低倍镜下取出，还可便于继续观察另一张玻片标本。

如果实验全部完成，先用清洁纱布轻轻擦拭整个镜体（切记：不包括玻璃构件表面），再将物镜转成八字形垂于镜筒下，以免物镜镜头下落与聚光器相碰撞。然后使镜筒下降至两物镜侧面与镜台轻触为止，并转动反射镜，使镜面与镜台垂直，方可放入显微镜箱内。

三、显微镜的维护

1. 必须熟悉并严格执行上述显微镜的操作步骤和规则。

2. 避免灰尘、试剂或溶液沾污或滴到显微镜上，如沾污了玻璃构件表面，应立即用擦镜纸擦拭干净，其余部位则应用清洁纱布尽快擦拭干净。

3. 玻璃构件表面比较脆弱，尤其是物镜、目镜和聚光器内的透镜比一般玻璃的硬度小，易于损伤，因此只能用专用的擦镜纸，不能用棉花、棉布或其他物品擦拭，更不能用手直接接触。擦时要先将擦镜纸折叠为四折，绕着物镜或目镜等的轴按一个方向旋转地轻轻擦拭。如不按上述方式擦拭，落在镜头上的灰尘很容易损伤透镜，出现一条条的划痕。为节约，擦透镜后的擦镜纸还可以用来擦反射镜。

4. 显微镜为精密仪器，随时都应小心使用，不可任意拆卸，遇有机件失灵或阻滞现象，绝不能强力扭转，应及时查明原因，排除障碍，以便适时修理。

5. 保持显微镜箱内干燥、清洁，取出和放回显微镜后，立即关闭显微镜箱，并适时更换干燥剂。

第二节　绘图技术、植物标本的采集与鉴定

一、绘图的要求与方法

植物学研究成果的表达形式除了有文字、照片、实物等，绘图常常也是比较简而易行的方法。学者必须掌握绘图技术：绘图是重要的实验报告之一，比文字记录生动具体，可以帮助我们理解植物的结构和特征。

植物学绘图有其自身的特点，它着重从研究问题的事实出发，强调科学性，在此基础上适当地注意艺术性的表现手法，是科学与艺术的产物。而艺术性绘图是从创作观点出发，

加以艺术加工，着重艺术性、现实性、思想性。

植物学徒手绘图的具体要求如下：

（1）首先要注意科学性和准确性。必须认真观察要画的对象，对目的物进行全面的观察，弄清各个部位的特征及比例，在目的物中找出一个适当部分作为"标准"。

（2）画图之前，应根据实验指导要求的绘图数量和内容，在图纸上首先安排好各个图的位置比例，并留出书写图题与注字的地方。

（3）先绘草图，用 HB 铅笔轻轻地在图纸上勾画出图形的轮廓，以便修改。

（4）草图经修饰后再绘出物像。正式绘制时要用 2H 或 3H 的绘图硬铅笔，按顺手的方向运笔。把上述轮廓描绘下来，再对细小的部分逐步添加。线条要一笔勾出，粗细均匀，光滑清晰，接头无叉和痕迹（切忌重复描绘）。

（5）植物图一般用圆点衬阴，表示明暗和颜色的深浅，给予立体感。点要圆而整齐，大小均匀，根据需要灵活掌握疏密变化，不能用涂抹阴影的方法代替圆点。

（6）图纸要保持整洁，图注一律用正楷书写，并要求用平行线引出，最好在图的右侧，必须整齐一致。

（7）绘图及注字一律用铅笔不要用钢笔、有色水笔和圆珠笔。

（8）实验题目写在绘图报告纸的上方，图题和所用的植物材料的名称和部位写在图下方。并注明放大倍数。

二、植物标本的采集和制作方法

从事植物分类教学和研究，必须要采集植物标本，而且采集合乎规格的标本，以便研究和鉴定之用。

要采集一合格的植物标本，必须注意以下几点。

（1）采集标本工具的准备　一般应准备的工具有：枝剪、较大的铁锹、小铲子、标本夹，采集箱、草纸、粗绳和塑料布，高度表和指南针，野外记录本、标本编号的号牌、小纸袋（备装标本的花、果和叶，以便细致观察用）、放大镜等。

（2）采集标本时应遵守的原则

①注意植物的产地及生长环境。标本的采集地点及生长环境是非常重要的。因此有必要详尽地注明该植物产于某省、某市或某县，尤其是小区域应详细说明，植物的生长环境，如高山、平地、河泽、溪谷、丘陵、荫蔽处或是向阳、背阳处，以及海拔高度等。

②应采集完整的标本。种子植物在分类学上的鉴定依据主要是植物繁殖器官的形态特征，重点是花和果实，因此采标本要尽量有花、果或至少其中之一，如果无花、果则一般不采，另外叶子也很重要，如有地下鳞茎等应该挖取。某植物如只有花，则以后可以补采同种的果实标本。

③注意标本大小。装置标本的硬纸，叫台纸，而台纸的尺度一般规定为 42 cm×29 cm，因而标本的大小，要以台纸的尺度为标准，较大植物（草本）的标本可折成 V 字形或 N 字形，若植物体过小也可多采几份压制。

④注意有花、果的标本。在采标本压入草纸中时，注意解剖一朵花，展示其内部形态，便于以后研究。开花的植物标本，注意随时记下花期及花的颜色；有果实的标本，记下果

期和果的颜色，因为压制标本后，往往颜色褪去会影响鉴定。另外，要使叶片有正面的，也有叶背面的（常2~3片）。因为标本干后再翻动则易断裂。叶有上、下面可以随时观察其毛被等特征；特别注意有鳞茎、根茎或块根等的植物，应该挖取它们连同地上的部分制成标本。

另外，当一些植物为雌雄异株或同株时，应尽量采集异株植物包括花在内。同株则分别采雌、雄花枝。蕨类植物必须采有孢子囊的植株，便于鉴别，寄生植物最好连寄主同采。

⑤其他。采集的植物标本必须有编号和详细野外记录，并在标本上有相符的标本号牌。

（3）野外记录 一般采集应有野外记录本，且其有一定的格式，如图1-2所示。

中国植物

中文名：_____

拉丁名：_____

科名：_____

地点：_____

环境：_____

海拔高：_____

习性：_____

植物高：_____胸高直径：_____

根：_____

叶序：_____

花：_____

果实：_____

备考：_____

采集者：_____采集号：_____

日期   年   月   日

图1-2 野外记录表

表内各项填写应注意的是生境，写森林、路边、草坡、河边等。习性，为乔木、灌木或草本等。植物高可以估计写，叶要记明上、下面颜色和有无粉质及毛多少等。花记明花色，果实记明颜色和形状备考，记述植物土名，当地利用情况或此种植物的特殊情况如树皮颜色、数量等。

（4）编号 在同一地区同一时间采集的同一种标本，如采集5枝，应编为同一号。每张标本挂一号牌。如同种植物在不同地区采集，则编不同号。一般号数采用连贯法，不论换何地方，号数连续下去，不能换一地又从头编号。

号牌上写明采集时间、地点以及采集人姓名，有时也记录一些其他的东西。凡雌雄异株植物分开编号，写明系同一种的雌株和雄株。

号牌的样式如图1-3所示。

采集号码：＿＿＿＿＿＿＿＿＿＿＿＿＿＿＿＿＿＿＿＿＿＿

地点：＿＿＿＿＿＿＿＿＿＿＿＿＿＿＿＿＿＿＿＿＿＿＿＿＿

采集者：＿＿＿＿＿＿＿＿＿＿＿＿＿＿＿＿＿＿＿＿＿＿＿

日期　　　　　　　　　　年　　　　月　　　　日

图1-3　号牌的样式

（5）压制标本的方法　采得新鲜标本回来后，最好立即整理压制，若因时间过于急促而不能立即压制时，亦可待至次日，但要把标本摊敞开来。压制时应对照野外记录。压制的标本每天换纸至少一次，在换纸时用镊子将标本上不平整的叶弄平，叶既有上面的，也应翻1~2片使其背面朝上。一般标本带回后，应转入厚夹中用绳子捆压，增加压力。天气好时放日光下晒，经5~7日可以干燥；如遇阴雨天，可用火烤或勤换纸。天南星科和兰科植物以及多数肉质植物营养器官不易压干，且易落叶，可将此类标本浸入沸水中一分钟左右，以杀死其外部细胞，使之易于失去水分而促使干燥。

标本干燥后应消毒，一般用升汞（氯化汞，$HgCl_2$）消毒，用毛笔蘸升汞溶液刷于标本上以湿透，再放于草纸上晾干。然后方可上台纸做成永久标本，并于标本右上角盖印"$HgCl_2$消毒"字样。

标本上台纸时，注意布局美观大方，尤应注意不使花或果离台纸边缘太近，因为太近了在拿取标本时易折坏。每张标本固定常用纸条穿缝反贴；做好后，可以用标本名签写上名字贴在右下角。标本名签格式如图1-4所示。

×××植物标本室

采集号数：＿＿＿＿＿＿＿＿＿　　登记号数：＿＿＿＿＿＿＿＿＿

科名：＿＿＿＿＿＿＿＿＿＿＿＿＿＿＿＿＿＿＿＿＿＿＿＿＿

拉丁名：＿＿＿＿＿＿＿＿＿＿＿＿＿＿＿＿＿＿＿＿＿＿＿

中文名：＿＿＿＿＿＿＿＿＿＿＿＿＿＿＿＿＿＿＿＿＿＿＿

采集者：＿＿＿＿＿＿＿＿＿　产地：＿＿＿＿＿＿＿＿＿＿＿

鉴定者：＿＿＿＿＿＿＿＿＿　日期：＿＿＿＿＿＿＿＿＿＿＿

图1-4　标本名签格式

野外记录可以整体保存，也可以取下来贴在有关标本的左上角。

三、认识和鉴定植物

学习植物分类学，特别是被子植物的分类学，重要的是对一些重要科或种的植物特征熟记及理解，认知植物前应掌握扎实的、一定量的形态学及分类学理论知识。有些植物根据形态能较容易地判断出属于哪个科。这样就可以找到该科查分属检索表，属查出后再查种，种查出后，再根据种的描述一一查对特征，如基本符合就可以定出种名了。但如一植物不知道是哪一科的，则可根据科的检索表，先查出科名，再接上述步骤确定是何种植物。

如果是在野外，查找参考书较为困难，则可以做好编号，写好野外记录带回住处查寻。

在鉴定某一种植物时，有时会感到鉴定困难，这时可以到一些植物标本馆，查找标本对照植物进行鉴定。在认识和鉴定植物时，还常常会用到一些参考书，在这些参考书中，最常用的有：《中国植物志》《中国高等植物图鉴》《中国高等植物科属检索表》及一地方植物志，如《山东植物志》《江苏植物志》等等。这些参考书对认识和鉴定植物都有帮助。

识别植物是一个由量变至质变的过程，只有通过不断地观察、接触、总结，才能最终认识植物、了解植物，学好、学活植物分类学。

第三节　显微制片技术

一、徒手切片法

徒手切片法是用刀片把新鲜的或预先固定好的或软化的材料切成薄片，不染色或简单染色，用水封片后作临时观察，必要时也可制成永久性玻片标本。本法简单、迅速，能够观察到植物组织的生活状态，非常实用，但缺点是不易切薄切全，厚薄不均，不能做成连续切片。徒手切片的方法介绍如下。

（1）材料先切成适当的段块，切片断面以不超过 3～5 mm，材料长度 2～3 cm 为宜，便于手持进行切片。软而薄的材料，如叶片可用马铃薯块茎，夹住块茎材料再一起切片。有的叶片可卷成筒状再切。坚硬的材料可用水煮，软化后再切片。

（2）切片时用左手拇指和食指夹住材料，并用中指拖住，并使其稍突出于手指之上，以右手执刀片，平放在左手的食指上，刀口向内，且与材料断面平行，移动右臂使刀口左前方向右后方滑行切片，注意切勿来回拉锯，并在切片过程中应用水润湿材料的切面和刀面，以免切面破损。如此连续操作，将切下的薄片用湿毛笔轻移于盛水的培养皿中。再用毛笔挑选最薄的切片，取出放在玻片上制成临时玻片观察。也可用 0.1% 番红水溶液染细胞核和木质化、栓质化的细胞壁，以区分细胞核与细胞质、木质部（主要是导管）和韧皮部。

二、临时装片法

临时装片法是用少量的材料，如薄的表皮、切成的薄片或粉末等，置在薄片上的水滴中，加盖盖玻片制成玻片标本，或选用甘油醋酸试液、水合氯醛试液等处理后观察。

加盖玻片时应注意先用镊子轻轻夹住盖玻片，使其边缘与水滴的边缘接触，然后慢慢放下，放平盖玻片，使盖玻片下的空气逐渐被水挤出而不产生气泡，以免影响观察。

三、石蜡切片法

石蜡切片是制作永久性玻片标本的方法，其原理是对不易切的薄而均匀的样品，利用石蜡渗入植物组织中，使组织在石蜡的支持下，用旋转切片机切，然后将切片中的石蜡除去，制作大量薄而均匀的连续切片标本，长期保存应用。石蜡切片制作步骤复杂，操作精细，时间长，不可能在一般的实验中学习和掌握。其步骤为：①取材和固定；②冲洗和洗脱；③透明；④浸蜡；⑤烘蜡；⑥包埋；⑦切片；⑧粘片；⑨脱蜡；⑩染色制片。

四、压片法

压片法是将植物的幼嫩器官，如根尖、茎尖和幼叶等压碎在载玻片上的一种非切片制片法。这种方法经染色后可制成临时片，也可经过脱水、透明等手续制成永久的玻片标本。此方法普遍适用于植物细胞遗传学等方面的研究，如染色体数目的检查。

以洋葱的幼根为例，制作步骤如下。

（1）取材　取洋葱鳞茎新生长出的幼根。

（2）材料的固定和离析　当嫩根长到 2～3 cm 时，在上午 10～11 点之间，或夜间 12 点左右，将距根端的约 3 mm 处剪下，立即投入到等量的浓盐酸和 95%乙醇配成的固定离析液中，经 10～20 分钟浸泡，取出放入清水中漂洗 10～20 分钟即可。

（3）压片　取离析好的根尖一个，放在干净的载玻片上，用镊子将根压裂，滴 2 滴醋酸洋红或地衣红染色，放置几分钟再盖上盖玻片，用铅笔将对准盖玻片的材料轻轻敲击，使材料压成均匀的、单层细胞薄层。用吸水纸吸取溢出的染液，即可在显微镜下镜检，如发现染色不够，可将片子在酒精灯上微微加热，如染液烘干，可补加。如染色较深，可加一滴 45%醋酸进行分色。

第二部分 药用植物学实验

实验一 植物细胞

一、实验目的

1. 掌握植物细胞的基本构造。
2. 了解分布于植物细胞中的主要后含物的种类及其形态特征。
3. 学习临时装片法及绘制植物细胞图的基本技术。

二、实验材料

洋葱鳞茎、马铃薯块茎、蓖麻种子、桔梗根、大黄粉末、半夏粉末、甘草或黄柏粉末、印度橡皮树叶或无花果叶的横切片、苍术根的横切片。

三、仪器与试剂

显微镜、载玻片、盖玻片、解剖工具、纱布、酒精灯、培养皿、擦镜纸、吸水纸、蒸馏水、稀碘液、水合氯醛试液、稀甘油、95%乙醇和75%乙醇。

四、实验步骤

（一）植物细胞的基本构造

1. 制作洋葱表皮的临时装片 从洋葱鳞茎上剥下一片肉质鳞叶，用刀片在其内表皮划一个小井字，使井字中央切割的小块长宽成3～5 mm。用镊子撕下井字中央这小块透明的内表皮，按临时装片法（参见本书第一章），置于载玻片上预先加好的水滴中，用镊子将其展平，然后将盖玻片盐水滴一侧慢慢盖下，防止产生气泡，用吸水纸沿盖玻片一侧吸掉多余的水。

2. 观察植物细胞的构造 在阅读显微镜的结构和使用方法后，将临时装片放在低倍镜下观察，注意洋葱鳞片叶内表皮为一层细胞，细胞为长方形或扁砖状，排列紧密，没有细胞间隙。移动装片（图 2-1-1），选择几个较清楚的细胞置于视野中央，换用高倍镜再仔细观察，注意识别下列各部分结构。

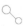

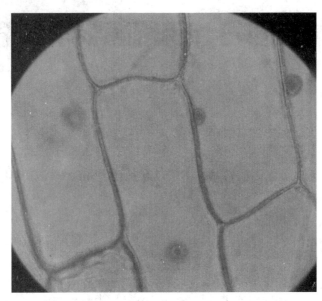

图 2-1-1　洋葱表皮临时装片

（1）细胞壁　为植物细胞所特有。位于细胞的最外层，比较透明。调节细调焦螺旋和虹彩光圈时，可见这层细胞壁实际为三层，其两侧为相邻两个细胞的细胞壁，中间是两个细胞所共有的中胶层（胞间层）。

（2）细胞质　为无色透明的胶状物，紧贴在细胞壁以内，被中央大液泡挤成一薄层，仅细胞两端较明显。

（3）细胞核　为扁圆球形的小球体，浸埋在细胞质中，贴近细胞侧壁的只能见其窄面，贴在细胞上下壁的可见其宽面。仔细观察，可见包在细胞核外的核膜，细胞核内有 1～3 个发亮的小颗粒，即核仁。

（4）液泡　位于细胞中央，占细胞体积的大部分。由于液泡内充满细胞液，所以比细胞质更透明。为了观察清楚，可取下制片，小心由盖玻片一侧滴加一滴稀碘液，由盖玻片另一侧用吸水纸吸水，使稀碘液渗入盖玻片下，几分钟后观察，可见细胞质被染成浅黄色，细胞核被染成较深的黄色。

（二）细胞器的观察

1. 白色体　用镊子撕取鸭跖草或玉米叶鞘的表皮，制成临时片，在显微镜下可见，细胞核周围有许多无色、球形的小颗粒，即是白色体。

2. 叶绿体　取藓类植物的"叶"（仅有 1～2 层细胞）制成临时片，在显微镜下可见许多绿色小颗粒，即为叶绿体。或取茶叶的横切片，观察叶肉细胞中的叶绿体。

3. 有色体　取番茄或红辣椒，去其表皮，取果肉细胞，制成临时片，在显微镜下观察，可见许多不规则的红色、黄色、橙色的颗粒，即为有色体（图 2-1-2）。

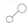

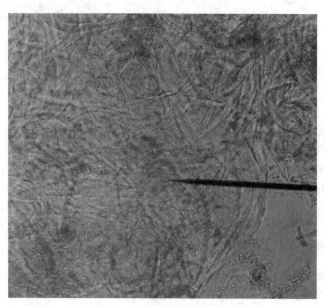

图 2-1-2　番茄的有色体

五、实验指导

（一）实验作业

1. 绘制洋葱鳞叶内表皮细胞结构图。

2. 绘制具缘纹孔侧面观简图，并简述纹孔类型及其结构特点。

（二）思考题

1. 为何细胞的各个部分遇碘液后会产生染色深浅或不染色的反应？

2. 在你的周围还能看到哪些形态的植物细胞？

3. 三种质体之间可以相互转化吗？

Experiment 1　Plant Cell

1. Objective

1.1　Grasp the basic structure of plant cells.

1.2　Understand the types of the main ergastic substances of the cell.

1.3　Study temporary slicing technique and the drawing skill of plant cells.

2. Experiment Materials

Bulb of Yangcong (*Allium cepa* L.), tuber of Malingshu (*Solanum tuberosum* L.), castor bean of Bima (*Ricinus communis* L.), root of Jiegeng (*Platycodon grandiflorum* (Jacq.) A.DC.), powder of rhizome of Dahuang (*Rheum officinalis* Bill.), powder of tuber of Banxia (*Pinellia ternata* (Thunb.) Breit), powder of root of Gancao (*Glycyrrhiza uralensis* Fisch.) or stem peel of Huangbai (*Phellodendron amurense* Rupr.), slid of cross section of leaf of Induxiangpishu (*Ficus elastica* Roxb.) or Wuhuaguo (*Ficus carica* L.), cross section of root of Changzhu (*Atractylodes lancea* (Thunb.) DC.).

3. Apparatus and Reagents

Microscope, slide, cover glass, dissector, spirit lamp, culture dish, lens paper, filter paper, distilled water, thin iodine solution.

4. Procedures

4.1　Basic structure of plant cells

4.1.1　Make temporary slides for onion scale leaf　Cut a slid of fleshy scale leaf from *Allium cepa* bulb, using forceps remove a transparent layer of the inner skin, cut into a piece 3~5 mm long, following instructions for temporary slide making (refer to chapter one), place sample onto an already prepared slide containing one drop of water. Smooth out the thin layer with forceps, then place another cover glass onto and slowly put down the cover glass to avoid bubbles. Lastly remove any excess water using absorbent paper.

4.1.2　Observe the structure of plant cells　After reading the construction and usage of the microscope, place the prepared slide under the scope. Notice that the inner layer of the onion skin is comprised of a single layer of cells. The cells are rectangular in shape, closely packed, without much intercellular space. Shift the slid and focus on a few well looked cells, switch to a higher magnification, to notice the following:

4.1.2.1　The cell wall　Cell walls are unique to plant cells. It surrounds the cell and

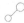

appears clear. When adjust fine adjustment and iris diaphragm, three layers of the cell wall can be seen, two layers of cell walls with a layer of middle lamella.

4.1.2.2　The cytoplasm　The cell is composed of a clear gelatinous substance, stuck closely to the inner cell wall, it is extruded into a thin layer by the central vacuoles, only the two end of the cell is clear.

4.1.2.3　Nucleus　The nucleus is a oblate spheroidal small spheroid, buried inside the cell body. Only the narrow side can be seen from the sides of the cell, the wide sides can be seen from the top of bottom of the cell. Also, 1~3 shiny dots can be seen inside the nuclear membrane, that is nucleolus.

4.1.2.4　Vacuole　Situated at the center of the cell, comprises most of the volume of the cell. Because the cell is filled with cell sap, the vacuole appears clear. In order to see the vacuole more clearly, carefully add a drop of thin iodine solution. Observe after a few minutes, pay attention that the cell now has a yellow tint and the nucleus is dark yellow.

4.2　Studying cell organ

4.2.1　Leucoplast　Tear a piece of epidermis out from leaf of *Commelina* communis or leaf sheath of Zea mays with forceps, to make a temporary mount and examine microscopically. Around nucleus there are a lot of achromatous and global grains, called leucoplast.

4.2.2　Chloroplast　To make moss's "leaf"(only 1~2 layers of cells) into a temporary mount, there can be seen a great deal of green granules under the microscope, which are chloroplasts.

4.2.3　Chromoplast　Peel off the epidermis of tomato or red hot pepper, and take the flesh of fruits cells to make into a temporary mount and examine microscopically.There are many anomalous red, yellow, and orange grains, which are chromoplasts.

Take up the scale leaf of *Allium cepa* or leaf epidermis of Commelina communis, spread it on the drop of water in the center of a glass slid, add 2~3 drops of alkaline purple, wait for 1~2 minutes, rinse three times and cover. When obserbe microscopically note that the nucleus, the cell wall and the mitochondria are all purple, whilst the latter showing itself like newly hatched silkworm.

5. Experiment Guides

5.1　Laboratory Assignments

5.1.1　Make structure drawing of endepidermis cells from the scale leaf of *Allium cepa.*

5.1.2　Make side elevation of the bordered pit, and point out the type of pits and their structural characters.

5.2　Questions

5.2.1　Each part of a cell acted by iodine liquid produces different color, from deep to shallow dyed or even colorless, then why?

5.2.2　Have you seen any other form of plant cells surrounding you?

5.2.3　Can three kinds of plastid convert mutually?

实验二 植物细胞后含物

一、实验目的

1. 学会识别细胞主要后含物的种类及鉴别方法。
2. 巩固临时装片法。

二、实验材料

马铃薯块茎、大黄粉末、半夏粉末、花生（果实）。

三、仪器与试剂

显微镜、稀碘液、水合氯醛、载玻片、盖玻片、解剖工具、培养皿、擦镜纸、吸水纸、蒸馏水、稀碘液、苏丹Ⅲ溶液。

四、实验步骤

（一）淀粉粒

刮取马铃薯块茎组织少许，加蒸馏水制作临时装片，镜下观察。可见有许多大小不等呈卵圆、类圆形的颗粒，即淀粉粒。注意观察单粒、复粒、半复粒的形态及淀粉粒的层纹、脐点的位置和形状（图2-2-1）。

观察后，于盖玻片的一侧滴加稀碘液一滴，并在盖玻片相对的一侧，用吸水纸吸水，使稀碘液逐渐引入盖玻片内，观察淀粉粒颜色变化。

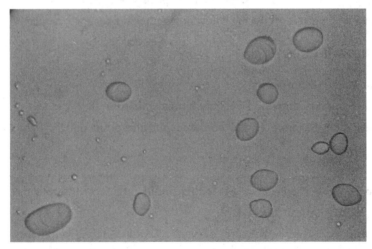

图2-2-1 马铃薯淀粉粒

（二）草酸钙结晶

分别取大黄、半夏粉末少许，分别放在两个载玻片上，滴加水合氯醛数滴，用解剖针边搅拌边在酒精灯上用小火微热2～3分钟。待玻片稍冷，再加甘油酒精一滴，调匀，加盖玻片，置显微镜下观察。这样的临时装片为水合氯醛装置，该操作过程称为透化过程。

（1）观察大黄粉末装片，可见星状或呈簇状的结晶，即为簇晶（图2-2-2）。

（2）观察半夏粉末装片，可见散在，但多集成束的针状结晶，即为针晶或针晶束。

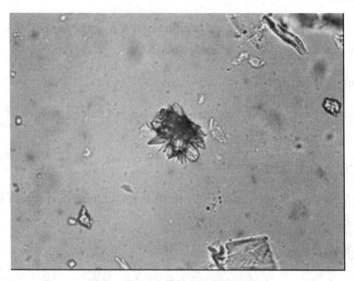

图2-2-2 大黄粉末中草酸钙簇晶

（三）油滴

取花生种子的子叶做徒手切片，并用苏丹Ⅲ溶液染色，观察可见被染成红色的油滴。

五、实验指导

（一）实验作业

1. 绘制马铃薯块茎中淀粉粒。

2. 绘制大黄粉末中簇晶、半夏粉末中针晶束。

（二）思考题

1. 为什么说淀粉粒、草酸钙结晶在生药鉴别中具有鉴定价值？

2. 你能说出已学过的植物细胞后含物的种类吗？

Experiment 2　Ergastic substances in the cell

1. Objective

1.1　Master the kinds, structural configuration of the ergastic substances in the cell.

1.2　Consolidate the method of temporary glasslide.

2. Experiment Materials

Tuber of *Solanum tuberosum*,　powder of *Rheum officinale*, powder of *Pinellia ternate*, *Arachis hypogaea*.

3. Apparatus and Reagents

Microscope, slide, cover glass, dissector, spirit lamp, culture dish, lens paper, filter paper, distilled water, thin iodine solution.

4. Procedures

4.1　Starch granules

Take up the tuber of *Solanum tuberosum*, and pare off to take a few turbid liquids with a razor blade, to make up a temporary water-mount and examine under the microscope. There can be seen many big or small oval, rounded shaped granules, which are starch granules. Note the following characters of starch granules respectively: shape of simple granules, compound granules or semi-compound granules and location, shape of striations or hilum.

Finally, place one drop of iodine TS in contact with the edge of the cover glass of the mount, and apply a strip of filter-paper to the other edge of the cover glass, thereby drawing some of solution under the cover glass. Note in the color of starch granules the changes observed under the microscope.

4.2　Calcium oxalate

Mount a few the following three powdered materials of *Rheum officinale, Pinellia ternate* in chloral hydrate solution (a few drops) respectively, heat gently above a alcohol burner while stirring occasionally (when doing this, move away the burner first), and if the solution becomes boiling, it should be removed to let it cooled off slightly and then heat again.

Repeat the above process three to four times, leave the glass slid to cool off slightly and then add one drop of glycerin alcohol, using the dissecting needle mix well, cover, wipe out excess of solution from outside of cover slip and examine microscopically.

This kind of temporary mount is usually called chloral hydrate mount and the process of making into suck into such mount is refered to as the hyaline process.

Observe the following characters of the crystals of calcium oxalate of each powder:

a. *Rheum officinale*: Astriod or clusters of calcium oxalate frequent, termed as cluster crystal.

b. *Pinellia ternate:* Scattered, or needle-like clusters of calcium oxalate frequent, termed as acicular crystal or raphides.

4.3　Oil Droplet

Cut the fleshy cotyledon from the seed of *Arachis hypogaea* into slices, then add several drops of Sudan Ⅲ TS, cover and examine microscopically.

5. Experiment Guides

5.1　Laboratory Assignments

5.1.1　Make sketch of the starch granules in Tuber of *Solanum tuberosum*.

5.1.2　Make sketch of clusters of *Rheum officinale* and raphides of *Ponellia ternate*.

5.2　Questions

5.2.1　The starch granules and calcium oxalate take on differential values in dried medicinal herbs, why?

5.2.2　Could you describe the sort of ergastic substances you have learned?

实验三　植物组织（一）

一、实验目的

掌握分生组织、保护组织、基本组织、分泌组织的形态、位置、结构及功能。

二、实验材料

洋葱根尖、薄荷茎、红薯块根、刺槐、山芋、天竺葵叶片、南瓜叶、柑橘果皮、姜根茎、当归根、松茎横切面、蒲公英根。

三、仪器和试剂

显微镜、水合氯醛、载玻片、盖玻片、解剖针、镊子、擦镜纸、吸水纸、蒸馏水、稀碘液、苏丹Ⅲ溶液、20%醋酸，1%番红水溶液。

四、实验步骤

（一）分生组织

1. 初生分生组织　取洋葱根尖纵切面制片，先置于低倍镜下观察，可以看到根尖先端的一个帽状结构，有许多排列疏松的细胞组织，叫作根冠。在根冠内方就是根的顶端分生组织（图2-3-1）。

在高倍镜下可以观察到细胞形状几乎等径，无细胞间隙，细胞壁薄，细胞质稠密，细胞核所占比例较大，且位于细胞中央，液泡很小（图2-3-2）。

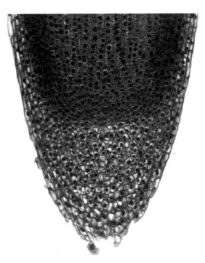

图2-3-1　洋葱根尖（低倍镜）

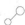

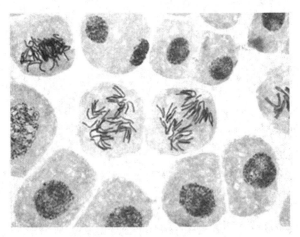

图2-3-2　洋葱根尖（高倍镜）

2. 次生分生组织

（1）形成层　取薄荷茎横切面制片，置于显微镜下观察，可见环状的形成层环，在维管束的木质部与韧皮部之间由一层细胞组成。注意形成层通常是排列整齐，紧密略呈扁长方形的细胞群，即形成层通常只有一层细胞。

（2）木栓形成层　取刺槐或其他树种的老枝，做徒手横切片，用 1%番红水溶液临时封片镜检，可观察到切片的边缘有多层扁平细胞，排列整齐且紧密，其中染成红色、细胞内无内含物的死细胞为木栓层。在木栓层内有几层颜色淡而扁平的细胞为木栓形成层，仔细观察其结构特点（图2-3-3）。

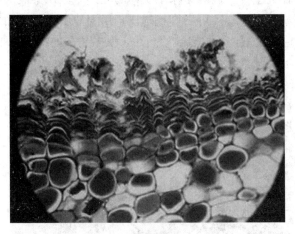

图2-3-3　木栓层与木栓形成层

（二）基本组织

取山芋块根，做徒手切片，镜检。可见许多近等径，多边形的贮存薄壁细胞。细胞间有间隙，细胞内可见许多颗粒，即贮存的淀粉粒（图2-3-4）。

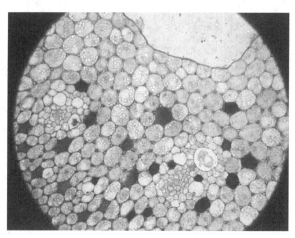

图 2-3-4 贮藏薄壁细胞

（三）保护组织

1. 初生保护组织 用镊子撕取天竺葵叶或南瓜叶下表皮一小片，用水装片，置显微镜下观察，注意表皮细胞形状不规则，彼此嵌合，无细胞间隙。在这些表皮细胞之间还分布着一些由二个半月形（肾形）的保卫细胞组成的气孔，保卫细胞含有叶绿体，而表皮细胞中则无。注意气孔的类型。

同时观察表皮上的许多毛茸，有先端锐尖的毛茸，为非腺毛，还有先端膨大成球状且具短柄的腺毛。

2. 次生保护组织 取厚朴树皮横切面切片，于显微镜下观察，可见最外侧有数层细胞，这些细胞壁厚，径向排列整齐，腔内无原生质体的死细胞，常染成深红色。这是木栓层细胞的侧面观。如果观察其顶面观，可去厚朴树皮，用刀片刮取其表面木栓组织少许，用水合氯醛装置，于显微镜下观察，可见多数淡黄色，呈多角形的细胞，即木栓细胞的顶面观。

（四）分泌组织

1. 分泌细胞 取姜根茎，徒手切片，用水装置，置显微镜下观察，可见散布一些椭圆形的细胞，细胞内充满黄色液体，该细胞即为油细胞，黄色溶液即为挥发油。滴加苏丹Ⅲ溶液，油液呈红色（图 2-3-5）。

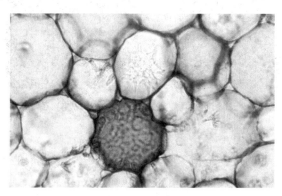

图 2-3-5 油细胞

2. 分泌腔 取橘皮横切片或徒手切片，置显微镜下观察，可见许多薄壁细胞围拢成圆形的腔隙，腔内有残余的细胞壁。有时还可以看到挥发油存在。这种腔内可看到残余细胞壁的分泌腔为溶生性的分泌腔（图2-3-6）。

取当归横切片，于显微镜下观察，可见许多由4～10个完整细胞构成的较小腔室，腔内有时能看到分泌物，即离生性的分泌腔。

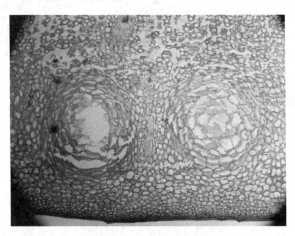

图2-3-6 溶生性分泌腔

3. 分泌道 取松茎横切片，于显微镜下观察，可见许多圆形的腔隙，它是由许多分泌细胞围拢成的管道，分泌道内可见树脂，分泌细胞完整（图2-3-7）。

4. 乳汁管 用刀片切取蒲公英根纵向薄片于载玻片上，滴加20%醋酸一滴，微热后，加苏丹Ⅲ溶液数滴，再微微加热，然后加盖玻片，在显微镜下观察，乳汁管内的乳汁呈红色，可以很方便观察乳汁管的类型及分布。

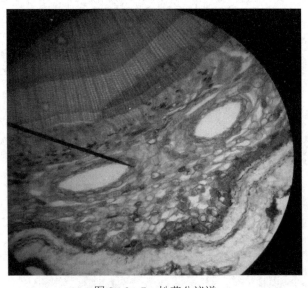

图2-3-7 松茎分泌道

五、实验指导

(一)实验作业

1. 绘制天竺葵叶表皮细胞及气孔、非腺毛、腺毛。

2. 绘制木兰树皮的木栓细胞侧视面和顶面观草图。

3. 分别绘制柑橘和当归根表皮中的分泌腔。

(二)思考题

1. 分生组织如何分类?它们有什么特征?

2. 什么是内部分泌组织?

3. 横切面上的裂生分泌腔与分泌道有无区别?

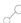

Experiment 3　Plant Tissue（Ⅰ）

1. Objective

Grasp the morphology, construction, location and function of a variety of tissues.

2. Experiment Materials

Root apex of *Allium cepa*, stem of *Mentha canadaensis*, root tube of *Ipomoea batatas*, leaf of *Pelargonium hourtorum* and *Cucurbita moschata*, bark cutis of *Citrus reticulata*, rhizoma of *Zingiber officinale*, radix of *Angelicae sinensis*, cross section of stem of *Pinus sp.*, root of *Taraxacum mongolicum*, *Sorbaria Kirilowii*.

3. Apparatus and Reagents

Microscope, glass slide, cover glass, dissecting needle, forceps, lens paper, filter paper, distilled water, thin iodine solution, Sudan Ⅲ solution, 20% ethylic acid, 1% safranine solution, brilliat green solution.

4. Procedures

4.1　Meristem

4.1.1　Primary Meristem　Place a slice of longitudinal section of root apex of *Allium cepa* under the low power, regard to a calyptriform construction at the head of the root apex constituted by many cells arranged loosely, which is called as calyptra, and to the inside of which is the meristem of the root apex.

Examined under the high power, cells are almost isodiametric with no intercellular space, and cell walls are thin with dense cytoplasm. Occupying large space, the nucleus locates in the center of cell with very small vacuole.

4.1.2　Secondary Meristem

4.1.2.1　Cambium　Take up the transverse section of stem of *Mentha canadaensis* mount and examine microscopically. The mount shows a distinct cambium ring, consisting of one layer of cells between the xylem and phloem in the vascular bundles. Note the cambium are often elongated and arranged densely and regularly.

4.1.2.2　Cork Cambium　Make a temporary mount of a transverse section of the *Robinia pseudoaccia* or other aged twigs with a razor blade, add 1% safranine solution, cover and examine microscopically. It will be found that the cork layer, composed of dead cells stained red with no ergastic substances inside of them, which among multilayer squamous cells arrayed

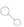

trimly at the rim of the slice. It can also be seen that the cork cambium is to the inside of the cork layer, which is composed of some layers of thin colored squamous cells. Examine structural features of the above tissue closely.

4.2　Fundamental Tissue

Cut the root tube of *Ipomoea batatas* into slices with a razor blade, and examine microscopically. The above mount shows that many storage parenchymas, which are nearly isodiametric, polygonal, and there are intercellular spaces between cells, within which they are plenty of granules, that are storage starch granules.

4.3　Protective Tissue

4.3.1　Primary protective Tissue　With the aid of a forceps tear apiece of epidermis down from a leaf of *Pelargonium hourtorum* or *Cucurbita moschata*, spread it on the drop of water in the center of a glass slid, When observed microscopically note that the epidermal cells have irregular forms tabled mutually with no intercellular spaces.

It will be found that between the epidermal cells spread some stomata formed by two lunate (kidney formed) guard cells, which contain chloroplasts. Note the structure of the stomata and their type(s) belonging to.

It can also be seen that numerous trichome occur on the epidermis. The non-glandular hairs are acute at the apex, and the glangular hairs are generally composed of a club-shaped stalk and a varicose bulbiform head.

4.3.2　Secondary Protective Tissue　Examine a permanent mount of transverse of the *Magnolia officinalos* bark microscopically. The above mount shows that the side elevation of the cork cells, which may be found near the most lateral aspect of the mount. The chief important characters of the cork cells are as follows: The cells are dead cells, deep-stained red, radial alignment regularly, the walls thickened, and inside the lumina there are no protoplasts.

Method for apical viewing of the cork cells is as follows: Using a razor blade, scrape some of the cork tissue down from the surface of the *Magnolia officinalos* bark, and to make into a temporary chloral hydrate mount. When examine microscopically, the cork cells present themselves as numerous faint yellowish and polygonal cells.

4.4　Secretory Tissue

4.4.1　Secretory cells　A slice of the rhizoma of *Zingiber officinale* mounted in water shows the following microscopical characters: Oil cells elliptical, scattered in parenchyma, containing yellowish oil drops (volatile), which are stained red when adding Sudan Ⅲ TS.

4.4.2　Secretory cavity　Examine the mount of the transverse section of cutis of *Citrus reticulata* under the microscope. Remarks: Several large cavities surrounded by some thin-walled cells, and this kind of cavity is formed by the dissolution of parenchyma, so the walls (sometimes even volatile oils) of some cells surrounding this central cavity still exist. It is termed lysigenous secretory cavity.

Place the permanent mount of the transverse slices of the radix *Angelicae Sinensis* under the microscope. It will be noted small cavities consisted of numerous 4~10 intact cells, which sometimes contain secretion. It is termed schizogenous secretory cavity.

4.4.3　Secretory canal　Under the microscope, the cross section mount of stem of *Pinus sp.* Possesses the characters as follows: Many secretory canals that contain resin are circular lacuna, composed of numerous surrounding intact secretory cells.

4.4.4　Laticiferous tube　Cut longitudinally the root of *Taraxacum mongolicum* into slices, select the thinner one to place it on a slide, add one drop of 20% acetic acid, heat gently, then add several drops of Sudan Ⅲ TS, and heat for a moment, cover and examine microscopically. Note the latex contained in the laticiferous tubes stained red, that makes it convenient for the observation of types and allocations of the laticiferous tubes.

5. Experiment Guides

5.1　Laboratory Assignments

5.1.1　Prepare the following drawings: epidermal cells, stomata, non-glandular hairs of epidermal cells in *Pelargonium hourtorum*.

5.1.2　Make sketches of the side elevation and apical view of the cork cells in the *Magnolia officinalos* bark.

5.1.3　Sketch the secretory canals found in cutis of *Citrus reticulata* and *radix Angelicae sinensis* respectively.

5.2　Questions

5.2.1　How to classify the meristem tissues? What characters do they bear?

5.2.2　What is the internal secretory tissue?

5.2.3　On cross section, does the schizogenous secretory cavity have distinction between the secretory canal?

实验四 植物组织（二）

一、实验目的

掌握机械组织、输导组织的形态特征、结构、体内分布及功能。

二、实验材料

薄荷茎、肉桂粉末、梨、苦杏仁、黄柏粉末、松茎、南瓜茎、向日葵茎、珍珠梅。

三、仪器与试剂

显微镜、水合氯醛、载玻片、盖玻片、解剖针、镊子、酒精灯、擦镜纸、吸水纸、蒸馏水、间苯三酚、水合氯醛试液、浓盐酸、甘油乙醇溶液、离析液、亮绿溶液。

四、实验步骤

（一）机械组织

1. 厚角组织 取薄荷或南瓜茎或向日葵茎，做徒手切片，用水装置（或水合氯醛装置）后于显微镜下观察，可见茎的四角处或棱角处的表皮之内，有一群细胞，其角隅处细胞壁加厚。因此，在三个细胞相接处加厚的部分就形成三角形，在四个细胞相接触的部分，就形成四角形。这即为厚角组织（图2-4-1）。

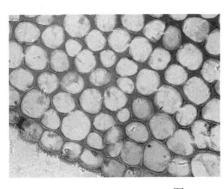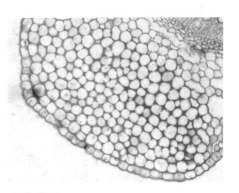

图2-4-1 厚角组织

2. 厚壁组织

（1）纤维 取肉桂粉少许，用水合氯醛装置，于显微镜下观察，可见有细胞呈长菱形（有些已断缺），细胞壁很厚，胞腔很小或看不清胞腔，这种细胞即为纤维。用吸水纸吸出玻片中的水合氯醛液，然后加间苯三酚和浓盐酸试液各一滴，放置片刻，加上盖玻片，置镜下观察，可见纤维细胞壁呈红色（图2-4-2）。

取黄柏（或甘草）粉末少许，用水合氯醛装置，于显微镜下观察，可见许多晶鞘纤维（图2-4-3）。注意仔细观察其结构。

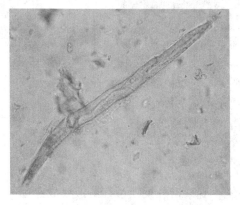
图2-4-2 肉桂纤维的晶鞘纤维

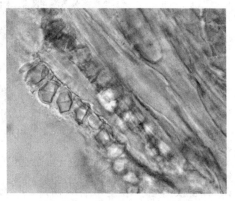
图2-4-3 黄柏的晶鞘纤维

（2）石细胞 用镊子撕取苦杏仁种皮一小片，以水合氯醛装置，进行观察，可见多数散列存在的黄色类圆形石细胞，其细胞壁增厚，细胞壁上可见许多纹孔。然后，如同上法吸水合氯醛，滴加间苯三酚和浓盐酸试液，注意石细胞壁的变化。

挑取少许梨果肉，压碎，用水装片镜检，可见一群群的细胞，其壁全面地增厚，细胞腔明显地缩小，细胞壁上层纹明显，并可见分枝状的孔沟（图2-4-4）。

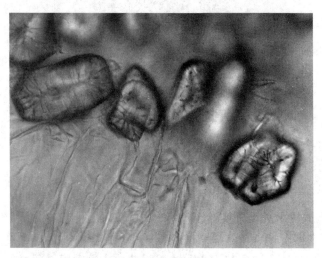
图2-4-4 梨的石细胞

（二）输导组织

1. 管胞 取松茎纵切片，于显微镜下观察，可见一些两端斜尖的长菱形管状细胞，即为管胞。在管胞壁上可见排列成串的圆圈，每个圆圈即是一个具缘纹孔，调节细调节器可见圆圈是三个同心圆（图2-4-5）。

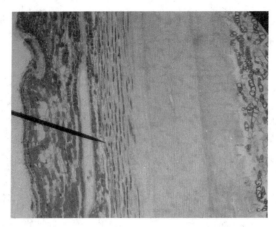

图 2-4-5　松木茎纵切面

2. 导管及筛管　取南瓜茎纵切片，于显微镜下观察，可见经番红溶液染成红色的长管状组织，即为导管群，在镜下尽量寻找各类型的导管。同时注意上下两个导管细胞之间是否有横隔。再于导管群侧观察经亮绿溶液染成绿色的薄壁性纵行连接的管状组织，即筛管群；在筛管中可看到原生质，是生活细胞，但无细胞核，在两个筛管节连接处能看到横隔，即筛板，其上有许多筛孔。在筛管的旁边，可以见到与筛管节的长短相近，而直径较小的长形细胞，总是伴随筛管同时存在，这叫伴胞（图 2-4-6）。

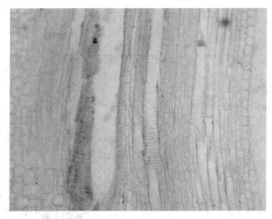

图 2-4-6　南瓜茎纵切面

3. 导管和管胞输导水分上升实验（示范）　取任何一种带叶并开白花的植物枝条，如珍珠梅等，将其插在盛有稀释的红墨水的烧杯中，一个多小时后，当红墨水沿着导管等疏导组织上升到叶片的尖端和白色花瓣中时，用手持放大镜观察红色脉纹，非常清晰，可以说明水分沿输导组织上升的途径及其在体内分布的状况。

五、实验指导

（一）实验作业

1. 分别绘出肉桂粉末、黄柏粉末中的纤维和晶鞘纤维。

2. 绘制梨果肉中的石细胞。

3. 绘制南瓜茎纵切片中的各式导管。

（二）思考题

1. 厚角组织细胞壁是初生壁加厚还是次生壁加厚？

2. 为何肉桂纤维的细胞壁在实验染色中呈红色？

3. 管胞和导管有何不同？

4. 如何利用伴胞在横切面上识别韧皮部？

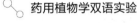

Experiment 4　Plant Tissue（Ⅱ）

1. Objective

Grasp the morphology, construction, location and function of mechanical tissue and conducting tissue.

2. Experiment Materials

Stem of *Mentha canadaensis*, steam of *Healianthus annuns*, powder of *Cortex Cinnamomum* cassia, *Pyrus sp.*, seed of *Armeniacae amarum*, powder of *Phellodendron amuranse*, stem of *Pinus sp.*, and stem of *Cucurbita moschata*.

3. Apparatus and Reagents

Microscope, glass slide, cover glass, dissecting needle, foreceps, spirit lamp, lens paper, filter paper, distilled water, phlorogluctional, concentrated hydrochloric acid, chloral hydrate test solution, glycerin alcohol, segregation liquid.

4. Procedures

4.1　Mechanical Tissue

4.1.1　Collenchyma　Cut the Stem of *Mentha canadaensis* or Stem of *Healianthus annuns* into slices with a razorblade, mount them in water (or chloral hydrate solution) and observe carefully under the microscope. The above mount shows that the collenchyma　composed of a group polygonal cells with thickened walls at their corners, which founded near the foursquare of the stem or underneath the epidermis at the corners of the stems. Therefore, if there are 3 cells attach to each other on their thickened walls, the collenchyma shapes triangular, and if there four cells, then the latter quadrangular.

4.1.2　Sclerenchyma

4.1.2.1　Fibers　Mount the powered *Cortex Cinnamomum* cassia in chloral hydrate solution and examine microscopically: Most of fibers are prismatic cells with thickened walls. And smaller or even unclear lumina.

Now blotting up the solution, add one drop of phloroglucinol TS and hydrochloric acid respectively, allow to stand for a moment, the ligmfied walls are stained red.

Mount the power of *Phellodendron amuranse* (or *Glycyrrhiza uralensis*) in chloral hydrate solution and the crystal fibers can be seen under the microscope, and note carefully their structures.

4.1.2.2　Stone cells　Mount a piece of the testa teared out from the seed of the *Armeniacae amarum* in chloral hydrate solution and examine microscopically: Most of the Stone cells scattered, yellow, subrounded, thick-walled and pitted.

According to the method of the above detection of lignified cell walls, test the stone cells. Pick up small amount of fleshes of *Pyrus sp.*, crush, mount in water and observed microscopically. The following distinguishing characters are apparent: The cells distribute in flock, the walls wholly and intensely thicken, and the lumina obviously reduce. The cell walls have apparent striation with branched pit canals.

4.2　Conducting Tissue

4.2.1　Tracheid　Place the mount of the longitudinal section of stem of *Pinus sp.* under the microscope, found that the tracheid is the long prismatic fistuliform cell with two bevel edges, strings of circles array on the walls of the tracheid, and each circle is a bordered pit. Fine adjusting, note the circle is composed with three concentric circles.

4.2.2　Vessel and Sieve Tube　Observed the mount of the longitudinal section of the stem of *Cucurbita moschata*. Microscopically, notice the groups of the vessels are long cannular tissue stained red by safranine. Note and record the types of vessels observed. Is there any transverse septum between the upper vessel and the lower ones?

Now, observe from the side of vessels, sieve tubes composed of thin-walled, vertical connected, cannular tissues stained green by brilliat green solution, contain protoplasm but no nucleus, which are alive. The sieve plate, which bearing many sieve pores, is the transverse septum located between the junctions of two sieve tubes.

Aside of sieve tubes, companion cells always go with sieve tubes, which are microscler, diameters smaller, and lengths similar with those of sieve tubes.

4.2.3　Water ascending through vessel and tracheid (Demonstration)　Insert a twig blossoming out white with leaves (such as *Sorbaria Kirilowii*, or *Hydrangea bretschneideri*, ect.) into a beaker filled with diluted red ink, and allow standing for more than one hour. Note under a magnifier, the red rat tails are very clear as red ink ascending to the top ends of blades and white petals through conducting tissue such as vessels, which demonstrates the ascending way of water through conducting tissue and its distribution inside the plant body.

5. Experiment Guides

5.1　Laboratory Assignments

5.1.1　Prepare the following drawings respectively: Fibers and crystal fibers in the powdered of *Cortex Cinnamomum* cassia, and in the powdered of *Phellodendron amuranse*.

5.1.2　Sketch the stone cells of fleshy fruit of *Pyrus sp.*

5.1.3　Make sketches of all sorts of vessels in the longitudinal sections of stem of *Cucurbita moschata*.

5.2 Questions

5.2.1 Is the cell walls of the collenchyma thicken in primary walls or in secondary walls?

5.2.2 Why do the cell walls of the fibers of *Cortex Cinnamomum* cassia stained red?

5.2.3 What is the difference between the tracheid and the vessel?

5.2.4 How to distinguish the phloem in the transverse section utilizing the companion cells?

实验五　根的结构

一、实验目的

1. 掌握双子叶植物根的基本结构。
2. 掌握单子叶植物根的基本结构。
3. 了解根的异常结构。

二、实验材料

蚕豆幼根、甘草根、百部根、何首乌块根、怀牛膝根。

三、仪器与试剂

显微镜、擦镜纸。

四、实验步骤

（一）双子叶植物根的初生构造

取蚕豆幼根横切面切片，置于显微镜下观察其初生结构（图2-5-1）。

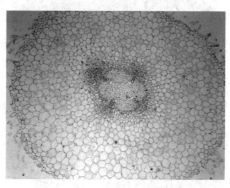

图2-5-1　蚕豆幼根及中柱横切

1. 表皮　表皮由1层细胞组成，细胞排列紧密而整齐，无细胞间隙，可看到有的表皮细胞突出形成根毛。

2. 皮层　皮层由多层形状较大的薄壁细胞组成，具有明显的细胞间隙。在显微镜下，可看到3个大的皮层细胞相邻处有一小的三角形区域，这就是细胞间隙。在较老的根中可看到有1～2层排列紧密的外皮层细胞。当根毛枯萎后，它们的细胞栓质化，起保护作用。在内皮层上可以清楚地看到被番红染成红色的凯氏点（或凯氏带）。

3. 维管柱（中柱）　蚕豆根的中柱鞘一般由1层细胞组成，但对着木质部束处常为二三层细胞。初生木质部具有4或5束（即四原型或五原型），也是外始式的。初生韧皮部在初生木质部束之间形成分散的束，在韧皮部的外侧可看到一些被番红染成红色的厚壁小细胞（韧皮纤维）（图2-5-2）。

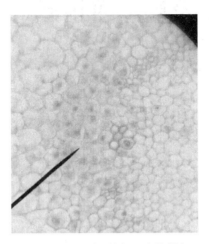

图2-5-2 蚕豆幼根及中柱横切

（二）双子叶植物根的次生结构

取甘草根或防风根观察，注意与蚕豆幼根初生构造有何不同（图2-5-3）。

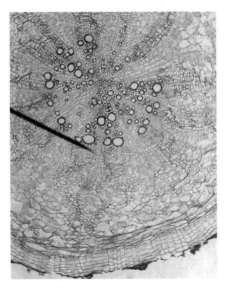

图2-5-3 防风根横切

1. 周皮 由木栓层、木栓形成层和栓内层构成。

2. 次生木质部 由形成层细胞向内分裂产生的细胞分化而来，位于初生木质部之外，其中可看到横切面上细胞腔较大的导管及木质部纤维细胞和木质部薄壁细胞。

3. 形成层 甘草根的形成层首先是由初生木质部与初生韧皮部之间的薄壁细胞恢复分裂能力形成的，然后逐渐向两边延伸，直至中柱鞘对着木质部束处的细胞恢复分裂能力，这时，形成层就在初生木质部和初生韧皮部之间成为完整一圈。在显微镜下看到位于木质部与韧皮部之间的几行径向排列得很整齐、形状扁平的薄壁细胞，看上去好似堆叠整齐的砖块，这就是形成层和形成层刚分裂出来的细胞。

4. 次生韧皮部 由形成层向外分裂产生的细胞分化而来，位于初生韧皮部之内，可看到筛管、伴胞、韧皮纤维细胞及韧皮薄壁细胞。

5. 维管射线 由形成层产生的一种横向排列的薄壁细胞组成，贯穿于次生韧皮部和次生木质部之中，起横向运输作用。在木质部的叫作木质射线，在韧皮部的叫作韧皮射线。

（三）单子叶植物根的构造

单子叶植物的根只有初生结构，没有次生生长。

观察百部根横切面，注意与双子叶植物根构造的区别，自外向内依次为：

（1）根被 为根最外的3～4层细胞，细胞壁上具致密的细条纹状加厚纹理。

（2）皮层 表皮以内维管柱以外是皮层，由多层大而薄壁的细胞组成，是除最外层（外皮层）外，细胞排列疏松，具较大的细胞间隙的这部分组织。

（3）维管柱 位于皮层之内，与蚕豆幼根相似，注意两者的区别。

（4）髓 中央具有发达的髓部，由许多较大的薄壁细胞组成。

（四）根的异常构造

1. 何首乌块根 皮部可见许多异心的维管束，为异常结构，均为外韧型。

2. 怀牛膝根 具有同心环状的异型维管束（图2-5-4）。

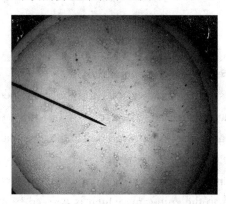

图2-5-4 牛膝根横切

五、实验指导

（一）实验作业

1. 绘制蚕豆幼根初生构造详图。

2. 绘制蚕豆老根次生构造简图。

3. 绘制百部根的构造简图。

（二）思考题

试比较单子叶植物根与双子叶植物根的构造有何不同？

Experiment 5   Structure of root

1. Objective

1. Master the fundmental structure of the dicotyledon.

2. Command the fundmental structure of the monocotyledon.

3. Know unusual structure of the root.

2. Experiment Materials

Permanent mount of *Vicia faba*, Permanent mount and root of *Glycyrrhiza uralensis* Frisch, Permanent mount and root of *Stemona sessilifolia*, *Polyonum multiform*, Permanent mount and root of *Achyranthes bidentate*.

3. Apparatus and Reagents

Microscope, lens paper.

4. Procedures

4.1   Primary structure of dicotyledonous root

Observe the transverse section of radical of *Vicia faba* mounted in balsam under the lower power, note from the external to internal, it is composed of three parts: Epidermis, cortex and vascular cylinder. Then change to the high power, notice the three parts characters in turn.

4.1.1   Epidermis   Locating at the extreme layer, it consisted of one layer of flat cells arrayed densely, with root hair bulging outwards. Are there any stomta or cuitcles here? Why?

4.1.2   Cortex   Interior to the epidermis which is derived from the ground meristem.They are consisting of a broad zone of parenchyma cells many of which contain starch grains. The cortex is divided into three layers: the middermis, storage parenchyma cells and the endodermis.

a. The middermis: Just below the epidermis, composed of 1~2 layers of thinned-wall cells which array densely and regularly.

b. Storage parenchyma cells: Composed of multilayer of thin-walled cells and often store starch, and arranged loosely.

c. The endodermis :The innermost layer of the cortex, composed of a layer of cells which are arranged tightly. Their radial and transverse walls are impregnated with lignin an suberin to form the structure called the Casparian Strip (Dot).

4.1.3   Vascular cylinder   Internal to the endodermis, composed of the four parts: Pericycle, primary xylem, primary phloem and thin-walled cells.

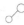

a. Pericycle: Close to the endodermis, constituted of one or more layer (s) of cells, thin-walled, and ranked tightly.

b. Primary xylem: Inside to the pericycle, radicalized formed.(In the radical of *Vicia faba,* composed of four tracts; and those near the vascular cylinder, called protoxylem; near the center of the root, called metaxylem)

c. Primary phloem: Alternate the primary xylem, cells are maller, thin-walled, multiangular. Found externally, thick-walled cells cluster, called phloem fibers.

Thin-walled cells: Some layers, bear the potential ability to generating.

4.2　Secondary structure of the dicotyledon

4.2.1　Periderm: Composed of cork, cork cambium and phelloderm.

a. Cork: Consisted of a few layers of flat rectangular thick-walled cells, rank radially and regularly, which are dead ones.

b. Cork cambium:One layer of thin-walled live cells bearing no protoplasm.

c. Phelloderm: A few layers of larger, thin-walled cells, which belong to ground tissue.

4.2.2　Secondary phloem　Composed of sieve tubes, companion cells (triangular or multiangular, dense cytoplasm); and thickened wall phloem fibers and thin-walled phloem cells.

Between the secondary phloem found inversed triangular phloem ray (thin-walled cells).

4.2.3　Cambium　Composed of 1~2 layers of cells, which elongate tangentially, flat, arrange densely and regularly, bear the ability to divide.

4.2.4　Secondary xylem　Inside to the cambium, occupy the main part in the transverse section, which include vessels, wood fibers and thin-walled cells.

Among the secondary xylem, there found xylem ray made up of wood thin-walled cells, which composed by 1~3 row cells.

4.3　Structure of monocotyledonous root

No cambium No cork cambium None secondary but primary structure!

4.3.1　Velamen　Composed of 3~4 layers of cells. Walls suberized and lignified with dense and fine striatins.

4.3.2　Cortex　Consisted of multi-layers of thin-walled cells.

Three parts: Exodermis;Endodermis: casparian strip and casparian spot;Middermis.

4.3.3　Vascular cylinder　Pericycle: Consisted of 1~2 layers of thin-walled cells, arranged tightly, founded near the endodermis.

Primary xylem: Line in the same way with primary phloem.

4.3.4　Pith　Composed of numerous larger thin-walled cells, and well developed in the center of Vascular cylinder.

4.4　Anomalous structure of root

4.4.1　Root tuber of *Polygonum multiflorum*

4.4.2　Root tuber of *Achyranthes bidentate*

Examine the section of root tuber microscopically, observe the difference between the two roots.

5. Experiment Guides

5.1 Laboratory Assignments

5.1.1   Make detailed drawing of the primary structure of radical of *Vicia foba.*

5.1.2   Sketch the secondary structure of root of *Glycyrrhiza uralensis* Frisch.

5.2 Questions

Compare the structural differences between the monocotyledonous root and the dicotyledonous root.

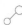

实验六 茎的结构

一、实验目的

1. 掌握双子叶植物茎的出生构造及次生构造。
2. 掌握双子叶植物茎的内部构造。
3. 了解双子叶植物及单子叶植物根茎的构造。

二、实验材料

桃幼茎、薄荷茎、桂枝、玉米茎、黄连根茎、石菖蒲根茎。

三、仪器与试剂

显微镜、擦镜纸。

四、实验步骤

（一）双子叶植物茎的初生构造

取桃或梨茎尖的成熟区做徒手切片或永久切片，置显微镜下观察，从外至内，依次可以看到以下几项。

1. 表皮层 位于最外层的一层扁平细胞，排列紧密，但有气孔存在，外壁常角质化，甚至形成角质层，有表皮毛。

2. 皮层 位于表皮层的内侧，是由多层细胞组成，靠近表皮的皮层细胞常形成厚角组织，用以增加幼茎的机械支持作用。薄壁细胞较大，具细胞间隙，靠近表皮的几层细胞常含叶绿体。桃幼茎皮层的最内一层细胞含淀粉粒，这层细胞称为淀粉鞘，但在有些植物中无淀粉鞘。

3. 维管柱 位于皮层之内，是由多个无限外韧的维管束构成的。但这些维管束排列成环状，束与束之间由髓射线分开。束中形成层明显。在高倍镜下仔细观察维管束各组成部分的细胞特点。

4. 髓和髓射线 位于茎的中心，由许多较大的薄壁细胞组成的部分为髓，髓部十分明显。由髓部放射地排列着多束薄壁细胞组成的髓射线，这些髓射线直通皮层。髓射线细胞起横向运输的作用。

（二）双子叶植物草质茎的次生构造

取薄荷茎横切片，于显微镜下观察，从外向内依次可看到以下几项。

1. 表皮层 同桃初生结构中表皮相似。

2. 皮层 位于表皮层的内方，由多层薄壁细胞组成。在茎横切面的四个角处，紧靠表皮层的一些皮层细胞形成厚角组织。皮层薄壁细胞排列疏松，靠近表皮的皮层细胞内含有叶绿体，能进行光合作用。无淀粉鞘的结构，内皮层不明显。

3. 维管柱 位于皮层之内，维管束是无限外韧的维管束，在横切面上呈环状排列，束中形成层与束间形成层明显可见，且连接成环。在四角处的维管束较大，是束中形成层活动的结果，而在两个较大的维管束之间，还可以看到2～4个较小的维管束，是束间形成层分裂的结果。在大的维管束与小的维管束之间仍可看到髓射线（初生射线），在较大的维管束中，可以看到放射线状的由薄壁细胞组成的维管射线。

（4）髓和髓射线 茎的中心存在较大而明显的髓部。髓射线也清晰可见。

（三）双子叶植物木质茎的次生构造

取桂枝横切片，于显微镜下观察，从外向内依次可见以下几项。

1. 表皮层 由一层排列紧密的细胞组成，表皮层的外侧可见角质层，在较老的片中表皮层已局部脱落或完全脱落。

2. 周皮 周皮是取代表皮起保护作用的次生保护组织，有些较老的片子，周皮完整，而有些较嫩的片子则周皮断断续续，中间与表皮层相间。周皮由木栓层、木栓形成层、栓内层组成。木栓层位于最外方，由多层厚壁细胞构造，细胞径向排列整齐，为死亡细胞。但在皮孔处不形成木栓层，而是形成许多薄壁细胞，这些薄壁细胞是生活的填充细胞。木栓形成层位于木栓层的内方，细胞扁平常为1～2层细胞，是生活的细胞，有较浓的细胞质及细胞核。栓内层位于木栓形成层的内方，由多层薄壁细胞组成，细胞质很浓，往往被染成较深的颜色。

3. 皮层 即初生皮层，位于栓内层之内，由多层薄壁细胞组成。桂枝片中，皮层细胞中有一环由石细胞群与纤维束相间连接成的环带。

4. 维管束 位于皮层之内，为无限外韧的维管束。次生韧皮部紧靠皮层，常被染成绿色，细胞较小，能观察到韧皮纤维。次生韧皮部所占比例较小。初生韧皮部应位于次生韧皮部的外部，但常常被挤压成颓废组织，不易辨认。形成层细胞扁平，排列紧密，位于次生韧皮部的内方。次生木质部在维管束中占较大比例，常被染成红色，可见口径较大的导管细胞分布其中。次生木质部可见年轮。初生木质部位于次生木质部的内方，也不易辨认。在次生木质部中，由许多由1～2列薄壁细胞组成的横向（径向）排列的微管射线，这些射线在到达次生韧皮部时变宽而形成喇叭形。

5. 髓部与髓射线 髓部位于茎的中心，较明显，由薄壁细胞组成，较初生结构中的髓部要小得多。髓射线由薄壁细胞径向排列，由髓贯穿至皮层（图2-6-1）。

（四）单子植物茎的构造

取玉米茎横切片，在显微镜下观察，由外向内依次可见以下几项。

1. 表皮层 位于最外侧，一层细胞组成，细胞排列紧密，无细胞间隙。

2. 基本组织 位于表皮层的内方，填充于茎的整个断面，是由许多大型的薄壁细胞构成。无皮层与中柱的分界。

3. 维管束 维管束散生在基本组织中，数量较多。是有限外韧的维管束，在每个维管束的周围有一圈紧密的厚壁细胞（纤维），称之为维管束鞘，在其内为木质部和韧皮部。仔细观察木质部和韧皮部组成细胞的特点（图2-6-2）。

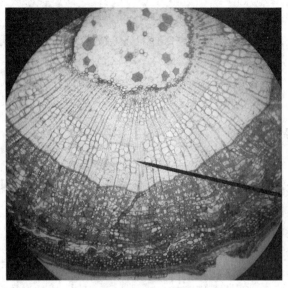

图 2-6-1 两年生椴木茎横切

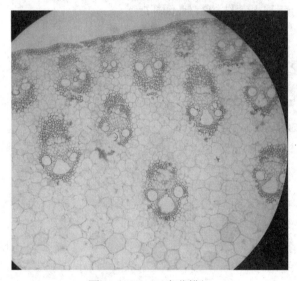

图 2-6-2 玉米茎横切

（五）双子叶植物根茎（地下茎）的构造

取黄连根茎横切面，置显微镜下观察，从外向内依次可见以下几项。

1. 木栓层 位于最外侧，由多层排列整齐，厚壁的细胞组成，常被染成棕红色。

2. 皮层 位于木栓层之内的多层薄壁细胞，在皮层细胞中有厚壁组织，皮层中还可见根迹维管束和叶迹维管束。

3. 维管束 位于皮层之内，成环状排列，是无限外韧的维管束。

4. 髓部 中央髓部明显。

（六）单子叶植物根茎的构造

取石菖蒲根茎的横切片，置显微镜下观察，从外向内可见以下几项。

1. 表皮层　位于最外侧，由一层排列紧密的细胞组成。

2. 皮层　位于表皮之内的多层薄壁细胞，皮层常占较大部分，可见叶迹维管束，内皮层明显。

3. 维管束　位于内皮层之内，由多数周木维管束构成。

4. 髓　位于中心，髓部明显，由薄壁细胞组成。

五、实验指导

（一）实验作业

1. 绘制出薄荷茎的结构详图（1/4）及结构简图。
2. 绘制出椴木茎的结构详图（1/6）及结构简图。
3. 绘制出玉米茎的结构简图及一个维管束的结构详图。

（二）思考题

1. 单子叶植物与双子叶植物的茎有何区别？
2. 双子叶植物根与茎的次生结构有何异同？
3. 双子叶植物的茎与根茎结构有何不同？

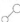

Experiment 6　Structure of Stem

1. Objective

1.1　Master the primary and the secondary structure of dicotyledonous stem.

1.2　Grasp the internal structure of monocotyledonous stem.

1.3　Know the structure of dicotyledonous and monocotyledonous rhizome.

2. Experiment Materials

Caulicle of *Amygdalus persica*, stem of *Mentha canadaensisi, Cinnamomum cassia*, stem of *Zae mays*, rhizome of *Coptis chinensis*, rhizome of *Acorus tatarinowii*.

3. Apparatus and Reagents

Microscope, lens paper.

4. Procedures

4.1　The primary structure of dicotyledonous stem

The plant material to be observed microscopically: Cut the maturation zone of caulicle apex of *Amygdalus persica* or *Pyrus sp.* of into slices with a razor blade to make into a temporary mount (or using permanent mount) and note the following characters inwards:

4.1.1　Cuticular layer　Possess epidermal hair and composed of the extreme layer of flat cells, which array densely, with stomata, wall keratinized or even form cuticle.

4.1.2　Cortex　External to the cuticular layer, constituted with multi-layer of cells. Cells near epidermis often form into collenchyma, which increase the mechanical support of caulicle. Larger thin-walled cells, with cellular interspaces, the ones near epidermis usually contain chloroplasts. In the cortex of caulicle of *Amygdalus persica*, cells in the innermost layer called starch sheath, contain starch grain, but in some other plants starch sheath absent.

4.1.3　Vascular cylinder　Within the cortex, composed of many open collateral bundle, which arrange annularly, set apart between them by pith ray, with apparent fasciculat cambium. Observe carefully under the high power the cellular characters of each component forming into vascular cylinder.

4.1.4　Pith and pith ray　In the center, pith is distinct, which is the part composed of numerous bigger thin-wallde cells. Radially arrange, consisted of numerous bundles of thinwalled cells, pith ray emit through the pith and reach the cortex. Cells of pith ray are functioned as transverse transportation.

4.2 Seconodary structure of dicotyledonous herbaceous stem

Examine the transverse section of the stem of *Mentha canadaensis* microscopically, and notice the following characters from external to internal:

4.2.1　Cuticular layer　It is very similay to that of primary structure of *Amygdalus persica.*

4.2.2　Cortex　Inside to cuticular layer, composed of multi-layer of thin-walled cells. In the four corners of the transverse section of stem and close to cuticular layer, some cortex cells come into collenchyma. The thin-walled cells in cortex range loosely, and the ones near epidermis contain chloroplasts capable of photosynthesis. No structure of starch sheath and no aooarent endodermis.

4.2.3　Vascular cylinder　Within cortex, open collateral bundles rank annularly in transverse section, with distinct intrafascicular cambium and interfascicular cambium, which connect to each other in the shaoe of rings.In corners, bundle become larger resulting from division of intrafascicular cambium, and between the two larger bundles there can be seen 2~4 smaller bundle, still found pith ray (primary ray), and between larger bundle there exist vascular ray (secondary ray), array radially, consisted of thin-walled cells.

4.2.4　Pith and pith ray　In the stem center, found larger and distinct pith. Pith ray is also very distinguished.

4.3 Secondary structure of dicotyledonous xyloid stem

Observed transverse section of *Cinnamomum cassia* microscopically and inwards:

4.3.1　Cuticular layer　Composed of one layer of densely ranging cells, found cuticle in the outside, and cuticulat layer fall of partially or even completely in some older plant materials.

4.3.2　Periderm　Secondary protective tissue which is the replacement of epidermis, in some older plant material, periderm is complete, but in tender one off and on and alternating with cuticular layer. Periderm consisted of cork, cork cambium and phelloderm. To the extreme outside, cork composed of multi-layer of thick-walled cells, which are dead ones, arrange radially and regularly. But in rengion of lenticel, no cork is formed, numerous thin-wallde cells produced, which are live complementary cells, instead of forming cork. Internal to cork, cork cambium constituted of 1~2 layer (s) of flat live cells, with dense cytoplasm and nucleus. To the inside of cork cambium, phelloderm made up of multi-layer of parenchymatous cells, with thick cytoplasm, usually dyed deep.

4.3.3　Cortex　Also called primary cortex, found inside of phelloderm, composed of multi-layer of thin-walled cells. Between cortex cells of transverse section of *Cinnamomum cassia*, there exist a ring formed by cluster of stone cells connecting with fasciculi alternatively.

4.3.4　Vascular bundle　Found inside of cortex which is open collateral bundle. Abutting on cortex, secondary phloem occupy less proportion of vascular bundle, often dyed green, with smaller cells, and there can be seen phloem fiber. Although primary phloem supposed to be lying to the external of secondary phloem, it is usually squeezed into decadent tissud and difficult to be distinguished. To the inside of secondary phloem, flat cambium cells rank compactly and tightly.

Occupying larger proportion of vascular bundle, secondary xylem often stained red, and vessel cells with larger caliber distribute in it, annual ring can also be found. Note carefully the characters of annual ring. Internal to secondary xylem, primary xylem is very difficult to be identified. Within secondary xylem, arrange transversely (radially), composed of 1~2 line (s) parenchymatous cells, numerous vascular ray broaden gradually to become flared when reaching secondary phloem.

4.3.5　Pith and pith ray　Lacating in the center of stem, pith is comparatively distinct, composed of thin-walled cells, and very smaller compared to that in primary structure. Array radially, consisted of thin-walled cells, pith ray penetrate through pith to cortex.

4.4　Structure of monocotyledonous stem

Mount and observe the cross section of the stem of *Zea mays* under the microscope, and notice the following characters inwards:

4.4.1　Cuticular layer　The outmost layer composed of one layer of cells, which arrange tightly with no intercellular space.

4.4.2　Ground tissue　Internal to cuticular layer, fill in the whole cross section of stem, constituted by a lot of large-scale thin-walled cells. There is no demarcation between cortex and stele.

4.4.3　Vascular bundle　Large amount of vascular bundle disperses in ground tissue, which is closed collateral bundle. Around each bundle, found a circuit of dense thich-walled cells (fibers), called vascular bundle sheath, and to its inside, found xylem and phloem. Observe the characters of constitutive cells of xylem and phloem carefully.

4.5　Structure of dicotyledonous rhizoma (underground stem)

Examine the cross section of rhizome of *Coptis chinensis* microscopically and inwards:

4.5.1　Cork　Locating outmost, composed of multi-layer of cells, wall thickened, line regularly, and often dyed red brown.

4.5.2　Cortex　Lying internal to cork, cortex composed of multi-layer of thick-walled cells, and cortex cells possess sclerenchyma, and there can be seen root trace vascular bundle and folial trace vascular bundle in cortex.

4.5.3　Vascular bundle　Lie within cortex, and arrange annularly, which is open collateral bundle.

4.5.4　Pith　In the center, pith is apparent.

4.6　Structure of monocotyledonous rizoma

Examine the cross section of rhizoma of *Coptis chinensisi* microscopically and inwards:

4.6.1　Cuticular layer　Lies in the outmost side, consisted of one layer of cells, which arrange compactly and tightly.

4.6.2　Cortex　Holding larger proportion, cortex composed of multi-layer of thin-walled cells to the inside of cuticular layer, and there can be seen folial trace vascular bundle with distinct endobermis.

4.6.3　Vascular bundle　Locate internal to endodermis, consisted of numerous amphivasal bundles.

4.6.4　Pith　In the center, it is apparent, composed by thin-walled cells.

5. Experiment Guides

5.1　Laboratory Assignments

5.1.1　Make detailed structural drawing (1/4) and sketch of stem of *Mentha canadaensis*.

5.1.2　Make detailed structural drawing (1/6) and sketch of *Cinnamomum cassia*.

5.1.3　Sketch structure of stem of *Zea mays* and draw detailed structure of vascular bundle.

5.2　Questions

5.2.1　What are the differences between monocotyledonous stem and dicotyledonos stem?

5.2.2　Depict the similarities and dissimilarities between dicotyledonous root and stem.

5.2.3　Depict structural distinctness between dicotyledonous stem and rhizoma.

实验七 叶的结构

一、实验目的

1. 掌握双子叶植物叶的构造特点。
2. 掌握单子叶植物叶的构造特点。

二、实验材料

番泻叶（或茶叶）、淡竹叶（或小麦叶）。

三、仪器与试剂

显微镜、擦镜纸。

四、实验步骤

（一）双子叶植物叶的构造

取番泻叶的横切片（图2-7-1），置显微镜下观察，可见以下几项。

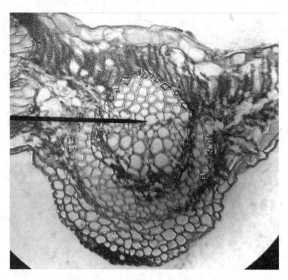

图2-7-1 番泻叶的横切面

1. 表皮 分为上表皮和下表皮，均由一层细胞组成，细胞呈长方形，是生活的细胞，细胞排列紧密，但有气孔存在，尤其在下表皮，气孔分布较多，组成气孔的保卫细胞较一般表皮细胞要小。有些植物的表皮上还可以看到各种毛茸。

2. 叶肉组织 位于上、下表皮之间，是较大的薄壁细胞。分成两部，紧靠上表皮的二层细胞为长柱形，垂直于表皮，细胞排列较紧密、整齐，细胞内含有较多的叶绿体，称为栅栏组织。靠近下表皮的几层细胞，排列疏松，有较大的细胞间隙，细胞呈椭圆形或类圆形，细胞内的叶绿体含量较少，称为海绵组织。在气孔的内方，常具有较大的空隙，称为孔下室。在主脉的上、下叶肉组织常常不分化为栅栏组织和海绵组织。

3. 叶脉　主要观察主脉的结构。主脉位于叶的中间膨大处。由维管束和机械组织构成。维管束是无限外韧的维管束，但形成层活动产生的次生结构有限。木质部位于近轴面，即靠近上表皮的一面，韧皮部位于远轴面，即靠近下表皮的一面，木质部与韧皮部之间有形成层。在叶脉处的表皮下常具厚角组织，尤其在下表皮处。随叶脉的越分越细，木质部与韧皮部的结构越趋简单。

（二）单子叶植物叶的构造

取淡竹叶（或小麦叶）的横切片，置显微镜下观察，可见以下几项。

1. 表皮　分为上表皮与下表皮，均由一层细胞组成，排列紧密，细胞外壁角质化，另外还有突起的硅质细胞。在上表皮中可以看到多个大型的薄壁细胞排成扇形，称为泡状细胞或运动细胞。

2. 叶肉组织　淡竹叶中同样分化成栅栏组织与海绵组织。但小麦等一些单子叶植物不分化成栅栏组织与海绵组织，而为叶肉组织。

3. 叶脉　由机械组织与维管束组成，维管束为有限外韧的维管束，无形成层。维管束的上、下方的表皮以内，通常可见到成群的厚壁细胞。

五、实验指导

（一）实验作业

1. 绘制出番泻叶的显微结构详图及简图。

2. 绘制出淡竹叶的显微结构详图。

（二）思考题

1. 在显微镜下如何判断茶叶的上、下表皮？

2. 双子叶植物与单子叶植物叶的显微结构有何异同？

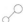

Experiment 7　Structure of Leaf

1. Objective

1.1　Thoroughly understand the structural characteristics of dicotyledonous leaf.

1.2　Grasp the structural characteristics of monocotyledonous leaf.

2. Experiment Materials

Leaf of *Cassia angustifolia* Vahl (or leaf of *Camellia sinensis*), leaf of *Lophatherum gracile* (or leaf of *Triticum aestivum*).

3. Apparatus and Reagents

Microscope, lens paper.

4. Procedures

4.1　Structure of dicotyledonous leaf

Examine the transverse section of Leaf of *Cassia angustifolia* Vahl under microscope:

4.1.1　Epidermis　Fall into the upper epidermis and the lower epidermis. Composed of one layer of cells respectively. The cells are rectangular, living, array tightly, and bear stomata, which have a far higher density in the lower epidermis than in the upper. Guard cells composing of the stomata are smaller than ordinary epidermal celts. In the epidermis of some plant, there can be seen a variety of trichoma.

4.1.2　Mesophyll tissue　Larger thin-walled cells, located between the upper epidermis and the lower epidermis. It is divided into two parts, the palisade parenchyma: consisted of two layers of cylindrical cells, usually directly beneath the epidermis of the upper surface of the leaf. The cells arrange tightly, perpendicular to the epidermis, and contain many chloroplasts; the spongy parenchyma: several layers of cells just under the lower epidermis, array loosely, bearing larger intercellular spaces. The elongated and cylindrical shapes of the spongy cells contain fewer chloroplasts. Internal to the stomata, there are usually bigger spaces, called sub-stomatic chamber. Usually, the mesophyllic tissues located in the main vein do not differentiate into the palisade and spongy parenchyma.

4.1.3　Vein　Observe mainly the structure of vein. Located in the bulge of leaf center, the main vein, made up of vascular bundles and mechanical tissues. Although the bundles are open collateral bundles, the secondary structures produced by activities of cambium are very limited. The xylem is adaxial, that is ventral, towards the axis, the upper epidermis, the phloem is abaxial, that is dorsal, away from the axis, the upper epidermis. The cambium locates between the xylem and the phloem. Under the epidermis of the vain, often there can be seen collenchyma, especially at the lower epidermis. The more division of the vein, the simpler the structures of xylem and phloem tend to be.

4.2　Structure of monocotyledonous leaf

Observe the cross-section mount of leaf of *Lophatherum gracile* (or leaf of *Triticum aestivum*) under the microscope:

4.2.1　Epidermis　It is divided into the upper epidermis and the lower epidermis. Consisted of one layer of cells respectively, arrange tightly, the cells wall keratinized, and bossed silica cells also can be seen. In the upper epidermis, there can be seen multi large thin-walled cells arranged in the fan shaped, which are called bulliform cells or motor cells.

4.2.2　Mesophyll tissue　In the leaf of *Lophatherum gracile* similarly differentiate into the palisade and the spongy parenchyma. However, most of the monocotyledonous plants like leaf of *Triticum aestivum*, differentiate into the mesophyllic tissue instead.

4.2.3　Vein　It composed of the mechanical tissue and the vascular bundles, and the latter are closed collateral bundles, with no cambium. Confined to the vascular bundles of the upper and lower epidermis, usually found clustered thick-walled cells.

5. Experiment Guides

5.1　Laboratory Assignments

5.1.1　Make detailed drawing and sketch of microscopic structure of Leaf of *Cassia angustifolia* Vahl.

5.1.2　Make detailed drawing of microscopic structure of leaf of *Lophatherum gracile*.

5.2　Questions

5.2.1　In the microscope, how to identify the upper and the lower of epidermis from Leaf of *Camellia sinensis*?

5.2.2　What are the similarities and the differences of microscopic structure between the dicotyledon and the monocotyledon?

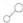

实验八　花与种子的解剖

一、实验目的

1. 熟悉花的组成。
2. 掌握花的解剖方法及使用花程式描述花的方法。

二、实验材料

刺槐花、凤尾丝兰、校园植物、蓖麻子。

三、仪器与试剂

体式显微镜、载玻片、镊子、解剖针、培养皿、擦镜纸。

四、实验步骤

（一）花的解剖

解剖前，应注意花序的类型，花的着生方位；苞片有无；花的对称性；合瓣花还是离瓣花；两性花还是单性花等。

如是新鲜材料，可放入培养皿中，先用解剖针将花按住，用镊子或另一解剖针自外而内层层解剖。如是干燥标本，应先在烧杯中加入适量的水浸润展开，然后解剖。

解剖时，应边解剖，边记录，一般为以下几项。

1. 花萼　花的最外部，由数片萼片组成。仔细观察，花的萼片分成几片，分离或连合，彼此间排列方式。

2. 花冠　在花萼内侧，由几片花瓣组成，分离或连合，彼此间排列方式。

3. 雄蕊　雄蕊几枚，排列方式，有何特点，花药的方向。与花瓣的关系。

4. 雌蕊　心皮数目、分离或连和，子房室数，胎座类型、胚珠数。其中心皮数通常根据子房室数、柱头数、子房壁上的主脉数综合起来确定。注意判断子房的位置。

（二）种子结构

种子可分为有胚乳种子和无胚乳种子。取一枚蓖麻种子观察其外部形态，注意下列各部。

1. 种阜　海绵状突起物，位于种子较窄的一端。

2. 种孔　为一小孔，被种阜覆盖。

3. 种脐　为一点状疤痕。

4. 种脊　种脐到合点间的隆起线。

5. 合点　位于种脊的末端。

五、实验指导

(一)实验作业

分别写出刺槐、凤尾丝兰的花程式。

(二)思考题

怎样判断心皮数目?

Experiment 8　Anatomy of Flower and Seed

1. Objective

1.1　Familiar with the constituent of flower.

1.2　Grasp the anatomic method of flower, and grasp depict of flower using the flower formula.

2. Experiment Materials

Robinia pseudoacacia, *Yucca glariosa*, campus plants, seed of *Ricinus communis*.

3. Apparatus and Reagents

Steremicroscope, glass slide, cover glass, dissecting needle, foreceps, culture dish, lens paper.

4. Procedures

4.1　Flower anatomy

Before anatomy, notice the following characters of flower: the inflorescent type, direction of flower insertion, whether bearing bract or not, regular or irregular flower, gamopetalous or dialypetalous flower, bisexual or unisexual or asexual flower.

If the material is fresh, then place it into a culture dish. Then, pressing on it with the dissecting needle, at the same time take it apart inward with forceps or another dissecting needle. If it is a dipping flower with bigger thin, weak petals, fill the culture dish with more water so as to let petals to unfold, then dissect it according to the above method. If the flower is picked off from dry specimen, put it into a small breaker filled with proper amount of water, heat it above an alcohol burner (heating time depended upon the quality of the material), then dissect it according to the above method.

Take notes, while dissecting a flower.

a. Calyx　How many sepals constitute a calyx, separated or connected? In what way do the sepals arrange between themselves?

b. Corolla　How many petals make up a corolla, separated or commissural? In what way do the petals arrange between themselves?

c. Androecium　Number of the stamen, way of arrangement, its characters, direction of the anther, relationship of between the stamen, and the petal.

d. Gynoecium　Number of the carpel, isolated or commissural, connate degree of the ovary and the receptacle, number of chambers in the ovary, type of the placenta, number of the ovule. To make sure the number of the carpel, usually the number of chambers in the ovary, the number of the stigma and the number of the main vein on the ovary wall should all be taken into account. Notion and identify the insertion of position of the ovary: superior, inferior, or half-inferior.

4.2 Structure of Seed

Seed can be classified into the albuminous seed and the exalbuminus seeds. Observe a seed of *Ricinus communis* in laboratory, notice its external conformity and different part of it as follows:

4.2.1 Caruncle Spongy vesicular aerifera, located in the narrower end of seed.

4.2.2 Micropyle One orfice, covered by caruncle, at the position where the radicle extended out.

4.2.3 Hilum A punctual scar, located at the of short radial of caruncle.

4.2.4 Raphe Ridging between hilum and chalaza.

4.2.5 Chalaza Located in the end of raphe.

5. Experiment Guides

5.1 Laboratory Assignments

Write out the flower formula of *Robinia pseudoacacia* and *Yucca glariosa* respectively.

5.2 Questions

How to estimate the number of carpel?

实验九　藻类植物

一、目的要求

1. 观察藻类代表植物，了解各类植物的主要特征。
2. 识别常见药用藻类植物，熟悉低等植物的一般特征。

二、实验材料

海带、蛋白核小球藻、石莼、甘紫菜、石花菜、海蒿子。

三、试剂与仪器

显微镜、放大镜、载玻片、镊子、刀片、解剖针、培养皿、擦镜纸。

四、内容步骤

（一）褐藻门

1. 海带　植物体分为三部分：呈假根状的固着器、柄、带片。是药材"昆布"的来源。

2. 海蒿子　藻体直立，多分枝，分枝有叶状突起呈线行，披针形，气囊与生殖托生在小枝叶腋间。

（二）红藻门

1. 甘紫菜　藻体呈薄膜状，遇水后，手摸有黏滑感，紫红色或淡紫色，全藻入药。

2. 石花菜　藻体扁平直立，丛生，紫红色或红棕色，羽状分枝4～5次，全藻入药。

（三）绿藻门

1. 石莼　藻体呈膜状体，由两层细胞组成，基部具有多细胞固着器，全藻入药。

2. 蛋白核小球藻　植物体为单细胞，很小，卵圆形或圆球形，壁内有1个近似杯状的载色体和1个淀粉核，细胞之内有1个细胞核。

五、实验指导

（一）实验作业

将藻类的主要特征填入表2-9-1中。

表2-9-1　藻类植物的主要特征

	植物体	营养方式	色素	世代交替	生殖器及生殖细胞	合子发育方式
藻类						

（二）思考题

低等植物有哪些特征？

Experiment 9   Algae Plant

1. Objective

1.1   Observe algae main characters.

1.2   Be capable to identify commonly used pharmaceutical algae. Gain common characteristics of elementary plants.

2. Experiment Materials

Haidai (*Laminaria japonica* Aresch); Danbaihexiaoqiuzao (*Chlorella pyrenoidosa* Chick.); Shichun (*Ulva lactuca* L.); Ganzicai (*Porphyra tenera* Kjellm.);Shihuacai (*Gelidium amansii* Lamx.); Haihaozi (*Sargassum pallidum* (Turn.) C. Ag.).

Instruments and appliances: magnifying glass, dissector, microscope.

3. Apparatus and Reagents

Microscope, magnifying glass, glass slide, cover glass, dissecting needle, foreceps, blade, culture dish, lens paper.

4. Procedures

Observe simple kinds of delegate plants, point out their main characters, and decide if their plants are saprophyte or gametophyte.

4.1   Phaeophyta

4.1.1   Laminaria japonica   The plant is divided three parts: the fixed organ of rhizome, stem and body band. It is the source of crude drugs Kunbu (Ecklonia kurome Okam).

4.1.2   Sargassum pallidum   Algae is erect and have lots of branches, branches have leaf projectings, which shape is linear or lanceolate. Air sac and reproduction branch lie among leaf axil of short branchs.

4.2   Rhodophyta

4.2.1   Porphyra tenera   Algae is flat membranaceous, meted water, feeling sticky and smooth, purple red or light purple red.Whole plant is medicinal materials.

4.2.2   Gelidium amansii   Algae is flat, erect, growing thickly, purple red or red-brown, 4~5 pinnately branching, whole plant is medicinal materials.

4.3   C hlorophyta

4.3.1   Ulva lactuca   Algae is flat membranaceous, and consists of 2 layers of cells. There is fixed organ of lots of cells at the base of the algae. The whole plant consists of medicinal materials.

4.3.2 Chlorella pyrenoidosa Algae is a small egg – round or round cell. There is a similar cup-shaped chromoplast and starch, and a nucleus in the cell.

5. Experiment Guides

5.1 Experiment report

Tab. 2–9–1 List the main characters of algae

	Plant	Nutrition	Pigment	Alternation of generation	Organ and cell of reproduction	Growing form of zygote
Algae						

5.2 Questions

Write out the same characteristics of elementary plants?

实验十 孢子植物

一、目的要求

1. 掌握菌类的主要特征，识别常见药用真菌。

2. 掌握苔藓植物的主要特征，识别常见的药用苔藓植物。

3. 掌握蕨类植物的特征以及石松亚门、真蕨亚门植物的基本特征，并识别常见的药用蕨类植物。

二、实验材料

冬虫夏草 *Cordyceps sinensis* (Berk.) Sacc.的标本及子座横切永久制片；伞菌 *Agaricus campestris* L.的子实体新鲜材料或浸制标本、木耳 *Auricularia auricula* (L.ex Hook.) Underw、银耳 *Tremella fuciformis* Berk.、灵芝 *Ganoderma Lucidum* (Curtis) P. Karst 的子实体标本，茯苓 *Poria cocos* (Schw.) Wolf.、猪苓 *Polyporus umbellatus* (Pers.) Fr.的菌核标本；石耳 *Umbilicaria esculenta* Miyoshi、松萝 *Usnea diffracta* Vain.等的腊叶标本；地钱 *Marchantia polymorpha* L.、葫芦藓 *Funaria hygrometrica* Hedw.的颈卵器和精子器的永久制片；地钱 *Marchantia polymorpha* L.、泥炭藓 *Sphagnum palustre* L.等植物标本；紫萁 *Osmunda japonica* Thunb.、海金沙 *Lygodium japonicum* (Thunb.) Sw.、石韦 *Pyrrosia lingua* (Thunb.) Farwell、槲蕨 *Drynaria fortunei* (Kze.) J.Sm 的新鲜材料；石松 *Diaphasiastrum veitchii* Thunb.、卷柏 *Selaginella tamariscina* (Beauv.) Spring、粗茎鳞毛蕨 *Dryopteris crassirhizoma* Nakai、肾蕨 *Nephrolepis auriculata* (L.) Trimen 等的腊叶标本。

三、试剂与仪器

显微镜、放大镜、载玻片、镊子、刀片、解剖针、培养皿、擦镜纸。

四、实验步骤

（一）真菌类

1. 冬虫夏草的标本观察 取冬虫夏草子座横切面在显微镜下观察，近表面生有许多子囊壳，壳内生有许多长形的子囊，每个子囊具有细长、多数横隔的子囊孢子（图 2-10-1）。

2. 子实体的形态观察 取伞菌的标本观察其外形，具有伞状或幅状的子实体，观察菌盖、菌褶、菌柄、内菌幕、外菌幕、菌环等结构。

3. 菌褶横切片的观察 徒手制作菌褶的横切片在显微镜下观察，菌褶两面有排列整齐的子实层。在高倍镜下观察可见子实层中的担子，紧密地排成一层，担子棒状、无分隔，顶端有个小梗，每个小梗上长有一个担孢子。子实层还夹杂有不孕的菌丝叫作隔丝（侧丝）。子实层的基部是由菌丝体组成似薄壁组织，叫作子实层基。在菌褶的两子实层的中间菌丝

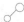

排列疏松，叫作菌髓。

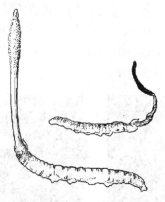

图 2-10-1 冬虫夏草

（二）地衣类

1. 叶状地衣 观察石耳，植物体呈扁平状，仅由菌丝形成的假根或脐紧紧贴在基物上，容易剥离。

2. 枝状地衣 观察松萝，可见植物体悬垂条丝状，成二叉分枝，先端分枝较多。

（三）苔藓类

1. 苔纲地钱的观察 植物的配子体为深绿色、二叉分枝的扁平叶状体，匍匐生长于地面上。在背面可以见到胞芽杯，内有胞芽。在有性生殖时雄株植物体上产生雄生殖托，雄生殖托圆盘状，7～8 波状浅裂，具有长柄。内生有许多精子器腔，每腔内有一个精子器。雌株上产生雌生殖托，雌生殖托扁平，9～11 深裂成指状裂片，两裂片之间生有一排颈卵器（图 2-10-2、图 2-10-3）。

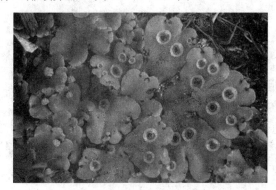

图 2-10-2 地钱示胞芽杯图

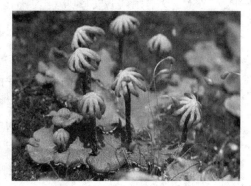

图 2-10-3 地钱示雌生殖托

2. 藓纲葫芦藓的精子器、颈卵器永久制片观察 略。

（四）蕨类

1. 石松亚门植物的观察 观察石松的腊叶标本，植物体有根、茎、叶分化。匍匐茎蔓生，二叉分枝。叶细小，螺旋状排列在小枝上，孢子叶穗常聚生于茎的顶端。用放大镜观察孢子叶穗，其孢子叶在孢子叶穗轴上，也是螺旋状排列。取石松孢子叶穗纵切片标本，置低倍显微镜观察，能清楚地看到每个孢子叶的叶腋处，有一个孢子囊。孢子囊内的孢子

大小一样，即为同型孢子。（图 2 - 10 - 4、图 2 - 10 - 5）

2. 观察卷柏的标本 茎多分枝，呈莲座状，具背腹性。叶子鳞片状，在茎上排列成四行，两行较大，两行较小。孢子叶穗生于枝顶。孢子叶的叶腋生孢子囊。孢子囊有两种，一个为大孢子囊，一个为小孢子囊，着生大孢子囊的孢子叶叫大孢子叶，着生小孢子囊的孢子叶叫小孢子叶，成熟的大孢子囊呈黄色，成熟的小孢子囊呈红色。

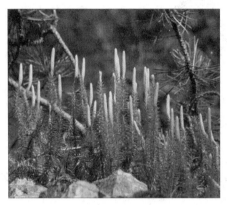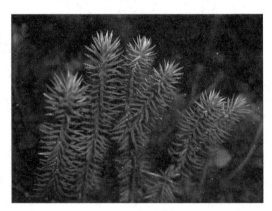

图 2 - 10 - 4　石松全株　　　　　　　　　　图 2 - 10 - 5　石松示孢子叶穗

取卷柏孢子叶穗纵切片标本，置低倍镜观察，可见大小孢子囊分别生于大小孢子叶的基部，大孢子囊内有四个大孢子，小孢子囊内有许多小孢子。卷柏孢子为异型孢子，与石松不同。

3. 真蕨亚门植物的观察 包括粗茎鳞毛蕨、肾蕨（蜈蚣草）、槲蕨、海金沙、石韦、紫萁等。观察粗茎鳞毛蕨及其他常见陆生真蕨的新鲜或腊叶标本的外形，它们的根状茎常有褐色鳞毛。根状茎向下生不定根，向上生大型复叶。注意叶脉的形态，孢子囊群着生的位置、形态，有无囊群盖等特征。

三、实验指导

（一）实验作业

1. 绘制冬虫夏草子座横切面图，并标明各部分名称。

2. 绘制葫芦藓精子器、颈卵器构造详图，标明各部位名称。

3. 绘制石松的孢子叶、孢子叶穗和孢子图，并标明各部位名称。

（二）思考题

蕨类植物是最为高等的孢子植物，主要体现在哪些方面？

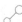

Experiment 10　Spore plants

1. Objective

1.1　Master the main characteristics of fungi and identify common medicinal fungi.

1.2　Master the main characteristics of Bryophytes and identify several medicinal Bryophytes.

1.3　Master the basic characteristics of Ferns including Lycophytina and Filicophytina and identify common medicinal Ferns.

2. Experiment Materials

Specimen of *Cordyceps sinensis* (Berk.) Sacc. and the permanent pieces of stroma, fresh materials of *Agaricus campestris* L., *Auricularia auricula* (L.ex Hook.) Underw, *Tremella fuciformis* Berk., *Ganoderma lucidum* (Curtis) P. Karst, *Poria cocos* (Schw.) Wolf. and *Polyporus umbellatus* (Pers.) Fr., specimens of *Umbilicaria esculenta* Miyoshi and *Usnea diffracta* Vain., permanent pieces of archegonium and sperm for *Marchantia polymorpha* L. and *Funaria hygrometrica* Hedw.; Specimens of *Marchantia polymorpha* L. and *Sphagnum palustre* L., fresh materials of *Osmunda japonica* Thunb., *Lygodium japonicum* (Thunb.) Sw., *Pyrrosia lingua* (Thunb.) Farwell, *Drynaria fortune* (Kze.) J.Sm; Specimens of *Lycopodium japonicum* Thunb., *Selaginella tamariscina* (Beauv.) Spring, *Dryopteris crassirhizoma* Nakai, *Nephrolepis auriculata* (L.) Trimen.

3. Apparatus and Reagents

Microscope, magnifying glass, microscope slide, cover glass, dissecting tool, foreceps, blade, culture dish, mirror paper, absorbent paper, distilled water.

4. Procedures

4.1　Fungi

4.1.1　Specimens observation of Chinese caterpillar fungus　The spores of Chinese caterpillar fungus invade insect larvae, spreading, destroy the interior of a worm, the worm become full of hyphae, mycelium form the sclerotium in the winter, the larva body head develop clavate stroma in the summer. Observe the cross cutting permanent pieces of *Cordyceps sinensis* stroma, near surface have many perithecia, there are many elongated shell endogenous ascus, each ascus have a slender majority across the ascospore.

Morphological observation of the sporophore　The specimens of the mushroom are observed, the mushroom has umbrella-shaped or radiated sporophore, meanwhile, the pileus, stipe, gills, universal veil, partial veil, annulus are observed.

The observation of transverse section of gills. The transverse section of gills is observed under the microscope, and the hymenium are arranged on both sides. Basidiums are visible in the hymenial layer under a higher power microscope. Basidiums are closely arranged in a layer. Basidiums is rod, no space, there's a little stalk at the top. Each stalk has a bearing basidiospore. The hypha is also interspersed with sterile mycelium (lateral filament). The base of hymenium is composed of mycelium, which is called a parenchyma. The middle mycelium of the two layers of the gills is loosely arranged, called mycelia.

4.2 Lichenes

4.2.1 Foliose lichenes   Observe *Umbilicaria esculenta*, the plant body is flat, the false roots or the umbilicus formed by the mycelium are tightly tied on the substrate, easy to dissect.

4.2.2 Fruticose lichenes   Observe *Usnea diffracta,* the plant body hangs filamentous, bifurcate branch, apex branch is more.

4.3 Hepaticae

4.3.1 Observe *Marchantia polymorpha*, make sure the following conclusions are correct : the plant's gametophyte is dark green, 2- branched flat thallus, creeping on the ground；on the back the cupules can been seen; in sexual reproduction, male plants produce male reproductive tots, male reproductive discs, 7～8 waves of shallow cleavage, with long handles; endogenous has many spermatozoa, each cavity has a spermatophore;the female reproductive tract is produced by the female plant, and the female reproductive tract is flat, and the numbers of finger lobes is 9～11, and there is a row of archegonium between the two lobes.

4.3.2 Musci Observe permanent production of spermatophore and archegonium for *Funaria hygrometrica.*

4.4 Fern

4.4.1 The observation of Lycophytina   Observe Lycopodium japonicum, plants have the differentiation of roots, stems and leaves. Stolons are creeping, bifurcated branches. Slender leaves spirally arranged on branchlets, sporophyll spike often clustered at the apex of the stem. Observing with a magnifying glass, the sporophylls are spirally arranged on cob of sporophyll spike, and sporangium can be seen in the axils of the sporophyll? It is found that sporangium could be seen in the axils of the sporophyll. The leaf axils of each sporophyll has a sporangium under a optical microscope. The spore size of the sporangium is the same as the spore.

4.4.2 Observe the specimen of *Selaginella tamariscina* (Beauv.)   Spring，determine if the following conclusions are true: the stem of the shape is lotus with multiple branches, with dorsal abdomen; leaf scales, arranged in four rows on the stem, two lines are larger, two rows are smaller; the sporophyll spike are born on the top of the branches;sporangium is born in the leaf axils of sporophyll, sporangium has two kinds, one is megasporangium, one is a microsporangium; the color of mature large sporangium is yellow, the color of mature

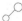

microsporangium is red.

Observe longitudinal section of sporophyll spike of *Selaginella tamariscina* under low power microscope, big and small sporangium is respectively born in the base of sporophyll. A big sporangium has four big spores, a small sporangium has many small spores. The spores are heterospores, unlike *Diaphasiastrum veitchii*. What is the significance of heterospore in the evolution of plants?

4.4.3　Observation of Filicophytina　*Dryopteris crassirhizoma, Nephrolepis auriculata, Trimen Drynaria roosii, Lygodium japonicum, Pyrrosia lingua, Osmunda japonica*. Observe *Dryopteris crassirhizoma* and other common terrestrial ferns, their rhizomes are usually brown. The rhizomes have adventitious roots and large compound leaves. Notice the morphology of the veins, the position and morphology of the sporangium, and the presence or absence of cysts.

5. Experiment Guides

5.1　Experiment report

5.1.1　Draw the cross section of the *Cordyceps sinensis* and indicate the name of each part.

5.1.2　Draw a detailed map of sperm and archegonium of *Funaria hygrometrica* Hedw. and indicate the name of each part.

5.1.3　Draw diagramssporophyll, sporophyll spike, spore of *Lycopodium japonicum* Thunb. and indicate the name of each part.

5.2　Questions

Why do you think that Fern is the most highest spore plant?

实验十一 裸子植物

一、实验目的

1. 掌握裸子植物的主要特征。
2. 识别常见的药用裸子植物,了解它们的药用部位及功效。

二、实验材料

油松 *Pinus tabuliformis* Carrière 枝条,雄球花、球果、松花粉装片;华山松 *Pinus armandii* Franch. 及红松 *Pinus koraiensis* Sieb. et Zucc 的腊叶标本;侧柏 *Platycladus orientalis* (L.) Franco,柏木 *Cupressus funebris* Endl. 带的新鲜枝条,具雄球花的腊叶标本等。

三、仪器与试剂

显微镜,擦镜纸,解剖针,镊子,放大镜,载玻片,盖玻片。

四、实验步骤

(一)松科

在解剖新鲜材料和观察腊叶标本过程中,注意采集记录及实物的下列特征:乔木、雄球花、雌球花,雄球花每雄蕊有两花药,雌球花珠鳞腹面具两个倒生胚珠、苞鳞与珠鳞分离(仅基部合生),球果木质,每种鳞有两种子,上端有单翅。

取油松枝条(图 2-11-1),区分出长短枝;短枝上的叶鞘宿存,着生针叶两枚。用镊子摘取黄色的雄球花,置放大镜下,见雄蕊多数,每雄蕊有两药室,用镊子和解剖针剖开花药,有粉状花粉粒,挑取少许花粉做成装片置显微镜下观察,能见两个气囊。雌球花生于新枝顶端,由多数珠鳞呈螺旋状排列等。取成熟的球果,辨别出一片种鳞(幼时为珠鳞),腹面裸露,着生两枚上端具翅的种子,以及种鳞上的鳞盾、鳞脐。(图 2-11-1、图 2-11-2)

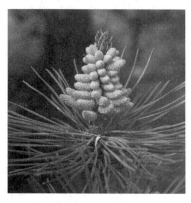

图 2-11-1 油松示雌球花

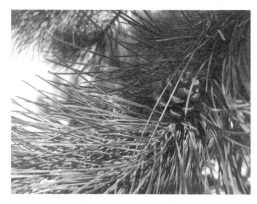

图 2-11-2 油松示雌球果

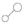

观察华山松，叶基的鞘早落，针叶五针一束，鳞脐顶生不明显，茎光滑，找出苞鳞和裸露的种子。落叶松属的红松，分辨出苞鳞与珠鳞是否分离。

（二）柏科

柏科植物为常绿乔木或灌木，叶对生或轮生，刺状或鳞片状，雄蕊具花粉囊 2～6 个，常多于两个，心皮的胚珠数目为 1～∞ 个，也常多于 2 个，木材分布树脂细胞。

取侧柏小枝观察：扁平，排成一平面，直展，鳞叶对生，放大镜下可见到叶背中部腺槽，球果椭圆形，有种鳞 4 对，种鳞反曲，其腹面茎部有 1～2 粒种子，无翅。

取柏木小枝，与侧柏小枝对比，描述与侧柏的不同：柏木小枝细长，下垂，种鳞尖头不反曲，中部种鳞茎部腹面还有 5～6 粒种子；用放大镜观察鳞片。总结与侧柏的异同点。

（三）其他裸子植物

观察苏铁、银杏、金钱松、三尖杉等植物的新鲜枝条或腊叶标本，了解它们的形态特征。

五、实验指导

（一）实验作业

1. 绘制油松的球果（雄球花和雌球花），并注明各部分名称。
2. 绘制松花粉图，并标明各部分名称。

（二）思考题

比较松科与柏科的不同点。

Experiment 11　Gymnosperms

1. Objective

1.1　Master the main features of gymnosperms.

1.2　Identify common medicinal gymnosperms, understand their medicinal parts and functions.

2. Experiment materials

Branchs of *Pinus tabuliformis* Carrière, staminate strobilus, cones, pine pollen slides; *Pinus armandii* Franch. and *Pinus koraiensis* Sieb. et Zucc specimens; *Platycladus orientalis* (L.) Franco, fresh branches of *Cupressus funebris* Endl with cones, specimens with staminate strobilus and etc.

3. Apparatus and Reagents

Microscope, wiping paper, dissecting needle, tweezers, magnifying glass, slides, cover slides.

4. Procedures

4.1　Pinaceae

During the process of dissecting fresh material and observing specimens, pay attention to collecting records and physical characteristics of the following: trees, flowers ♀, flowers ♂, each stamen with two anthers, the front side of female cone bead scales with two inverted ovule, bract scale and bead scale separate (base connate only), cone wood, there are two seeds each scale, the top has a single wing.

Distinguish the long and short branch of *Pinus tabuliformis* according to the length of the branches. The leaf sheath on the short branch is persistent and has two slender, soft needleleaves. Use tweezers to gather the yellow spikes from the sections of male cone and see under a magnifying glass, many stamens can be seen. Each stamen has two chambers. And then open anther with tweezers and anatomical needle. Powdery pollen grains are found, and then pick a small piece of sample under a microscope, two airbags (teaching) can be seen. The female cones born in the top of the new branch and many beads scales spirally arranged. Ascale (as pearl scales) can be seen from mature cone, ventral surfaces exposed, with two upper wing of the seed (note that understanding the characteristics of gymnosperms), appearance of scale shield and scales navel.

Observe the plant of *Pinus armandii*, the sheath at the base of a leaf fell off early,　five pin shaped leaves gather together. The scale umbilicus is not obvious, the stem is smooth, and the

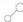

seed scales and the exposed seeds should be found. Observe *Pinus koraiensis,* and then distinguish whether the bractsare separated from the scales.

4.2 Cupressaceae

Evergreen trees, shrubs, phyllotaxis opposite or verticillate, leaves are spiny or scaly, stamens with 2 ~ 6 anthers sac, often more than two, one and more ovules, and often more than 2, resin cells in the wood.

Watch branchlets of *Platycladus orientalis*: determine the following conclusions whether are accurate: the plant is flat, arranged in a plane, heap, leaf opposite, back gland of the middle is visible under a magnifying glass, elliptic cone, 4 scales, scales contrary flexure, the front of stem has 1 ~ 2 seeds and stem wingless.

Observe branchlets of *Cupressus funebris*, compared with *Platycladus orientalis*, branchlets of *Cupressus funebris* are slender, sagging, a scaly tip is not an anticurvature, 5 ~ 6 seeds are distributed on the front of central bulb. Observe the scales with a magnifying glass in order to find out the difference between *Cupressus funebris* and *Platycladus orientalis*.

4.3 Other gymnosperms

Observe the fresh branches or specimen of *Cycas revoluta, Ginkgo biloba, Pseudolarix amabilisgingko, Cephalotaxus fortune* in order to learn their morphological characteristics.

5. Experiment Guides

5.1 Laboratory Assignments

5.1.1 Draw a cone of *Pinus tabuliformis* (staminate strobilus and female cone) and indicate the name of each part.

5.1.2 Draw diagram of *Pinus tabuliformis* pollens and indicate the name of each part.

5.2 Questions

Compare the differences between Pinaceae and Cupressaceae.

实验十二 蓼科 Polygonaceae、十字花科 Brassicaceae（Cruciferae）、蔷薇科 Rosaceae

一、实验目的

1. 掌握蓼科、十字花科、蔷薇科植物花部的主要特征。
2. 掌握蔷薇科四亚科的主要特征。
3. 学会使用检索表，并会编写出简单的检索表。
4. 识别各科代表的药用植物。

二、实验材料

齿果酸模 *Rumex dentatus*，油菜 *Brassica chinensis*，三裂绣线菊 *Spiraea trilobeta* Lindl.，多花蔷薇 *Rosa multiflora* Thunb.，桃花 *Prunus persica* L.，贴梗海棠 *Chaenomeles spinosa* Nakai.。另外有校园植物及若干植物标本：何首乌、大黄、大青叶等。

三、仪器与试剂

显微镜、放大镜、载玻片、镊子、刀片、解剖针、培养皿、擦镜纸。

四、实验步骤

（一）蓼科

取齿果酸模（或何首乌等）植物，观察其植物形态（图2-12-1、图2-12-2），特别注意其单叶互生，具膜质的托叶鞘（图2-12-3），茎节常膨大等明显特征。取其花于解剖镜下，

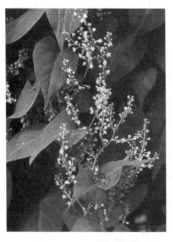
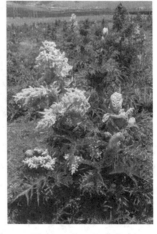

图2-12-1 何首乌　　　　　图2-12-2 大黄

边解剖边观察，花被片 6，两轮。内轮花被在结果时增大，有明显网纹，边缘通常有不整齐的针刺状齿 4～5 对，全部有瘤状突起；雄蕊 6；子房三棱形，1 室，子房上位，花柱 3，柱头流苏状，有基生胚珠 1 枚。

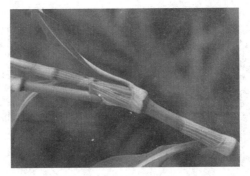

图 2-12-3 托叶鞘

（二）十字花科

观察校园中的十字花科植物，注意它们的花冠是怎样排列的？何种花序？雄蕊什么类型？果实的类型是哪一种？根据学过的知识，尝试鉴定一种教师提供的植物是属于哪一科的。

取油菜花于解剖镜下解剖并观察：可见萼片 4，仔细观察萼片是几轮着生的？花瓣 4，十字形排列；雄蕊为四强雄蕊；子房上位，心皮 2，合生，由假隔膜分为 2 室，侧膜胎座。胚珠多数（图 2-12-4、图 2-12-5）。

观察所提供的蜡叶标本，通过仔细的观察、比较，总结出蓼科、十字花科的基本特征。

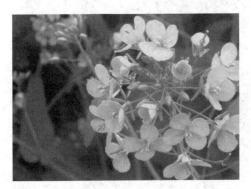

图 2-12-4 油菜

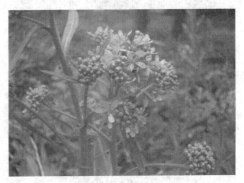

图 2-12-5 大青叶

（三）蔷薇科

蔷薇科四亚科检索表

1. 果实开裂的蓇葖果，稀为蒴果；心皮 1～5（～12），分离或连合，每心皮有 2 至多枚胚珠；托叶有或无 ……………………………………（1）绣线菊亚科

1. 果实不开裂，具托叶

  2. 子房上位。

    3. 心皮多数，生于膨大的花托上，每心皮有 1～2 枚胚珠；果实瘦果，稀为核果；

复叶，或为单叶……………………………………………………………………（2）蔷薇亚科

　　3. 心皮常为 1 个，少数 2 或 5 个，核果，萼片常脱落，单叶具托叶 （3）梅亚科

　　2. 子房下位或半下位：心皮 2～5，多数与杯状花托内壁连合，果实为梨果（假果）

………………………………………………………………………………………（4）梨亚科

　　仔细观察、解剖三裂绣线菊、多花蔷薇、桃花、贴梗海棠的植物形态及花。

　　三裂绣线菊，花白色，萼片 5，花瓣 5，雄蕊多数，心皮 5，分离，子房上位。

　　多花蔷薇，花粉白色，萼片 5，花瓣 5，雄蕊多数，心皮多数，分离，子房上位。

　　桃花，花桃红色，萼片 5，花瓣 5，雄蕊多数，子房上位，心皮 1 枚，1 室 2 胚珠。

　　贴梗海棠，花粉红色，萼片 5，花瓣 5，雄蕊多数，子房下位，心皮 5，合生，5 室，
每室胚珠多数（图 2-12-6）。

　　以上四种植物分别属于哪一个亚科？

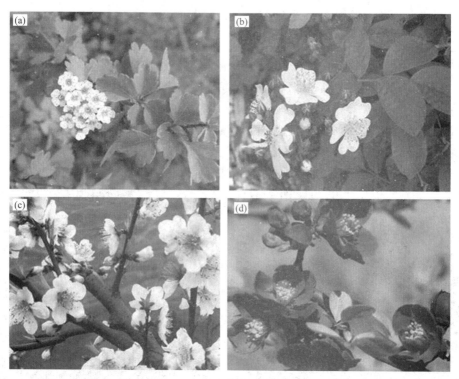

图 2-12-6　三裂绣线菊（a）、多花蔷薇（b）、桃花（c）、贴梗海棠（d）

五、实验指导

（一）实验作业

1. 写出齿果酸模的花程式，并绘出花图式。

2. 写出油菜的花程式，并绘出花图式。

3. 写出三裂绣线菊、多花蔷薇、桃花、贴梗海棠的花程式，并绘多花蔷薇、贴梗海棠
的花图式。

4. 检索蔷薇科的植物分属于哪个亚科。

(二)思考题

1. 齿果酸模的哪些特征代表蓼科的特征？

2. 十字花科有何特征？

3. 蔷薇科四亚科有何区别？

4. 试着用检索表检索一个未知植物。

Experiment 12　Polygonaceae, Brassicaceae (Cruciferae), Rosaceae

1. Objective

1.1　Seize the prirmary characters of plant flower in Polygonaceae, Brassicaceae and Rosaceae respectively.

1.2　Grasp the main characters of the four subfamilies in Rosaceae.

1.3　Know how to use the identification key, and learn to write simple key.

1.4　Understand the representative medicinal plants in each family.

2. Experiment Materials

Rumex dentatus, *Brassica chinensis*, *Spiraea trilobeta* Lindl., *Rosa multiflora* Thunb., *Prunus persica* L., *Chaenomeles spinosa* Nakai. Besides, there are some herbarium sheets, campus plants and other plant species such as: *Polygonum multiflorum* Thunb., *Rheum officinale* Baill., *Isatis indigotica* Fort., ect.

3. Apparatus and Reagents

Microscope, magnifying glass, glass slide, cover glass, dissecting needle, forceps, blade, culture dish, lens paper.

4. Procedures

4.1　Polygonaceae

Pick up *Rumex dentatus*., and examine the plant configuration, pay special attention to the evident characters as follows: single leaf alternate, leaves with nodal membranaceous ocrea, nodes often bulged, dissect flower of *Rumex dentatus*, and observe under the anatomical lens, found that perianth 6, 2 whorled, just think is it a simple flower or double perianth flower, why?

The inner perianth augments when bearing fruit, with visible reticulate pattern, 4~5 paired irregular needle-like teeth usually occur on the margin of perianth, nodular prominence present in all the perianth; stamens 6, ovary prismatic, superior, with single loculus containing a single basal ovule, styles 3, stigma fringe-like.

4.2　Brassicaceae

Careful inspection of plants of Brassica ceae in the campus, and give your attention to such problems as in what way do their corollas arranged, which inflorescence do they attribute to, what type do their androcium belong to, and to which kind do their fruit pertain?

Judging by the knowledge you have learned, try to identify the plant provided by teacher to confirm its family.

Pick up a flower of *Brassica chinensis*, dissect and observe under the anatomical lens, it is found: sepals 4(examine for sepals, how many whorls do they inserted?), petals 4, arranged in or forming a cross; tetradynamous stamen, ovary superior, 2-carpellate, syncarpous. Ovary divided into 2 locule by false dissepiment, with parietal placenta and numerous ovules.

Taking stock of provided herbarium sheets, sum up the fundamental characters of Polygonaceae, Brassicaceae respectively, through careful observation and compare.

4.3 Rosaceae

Identification key of the four subfamilies in Rosaceae.

1. Fruit a dehiscent follicle, seldom a capsule; carpels1－5(－12), apocarpous or syncarpous, 2 to numerous ovules of each carpel; stipules present or absent ···(1) Spiraeoideae

 1. Indehiscent fruit, bearing stipules

  2. Ovary superior

   3. Numerous carpels, occurred from the swollen receptacle, and each carpel contains 1－2 ovules; fruit a achene, seldom a drupe; leaves compound, or simple ··· (2) Rosoideae

   3. Carpels usually 1, seldom 2 or 5, fruit a drupe, sepals usually fall off, leaves simple with stipules ·· (3) Prunoideae

  2. Ovary inferior or half－inferior: carpels 2－5, usually inosculated with cup－like receptacles, fruit a pome··· (4) Maloideae

Dissect and observe carefully the plant configuration and flower of *Spiraea trilobata* Lindl., *Rosa multiflora* Thunb., *Prunus persica* L., *Chaenomeles spinosa* Nakai. respectively.

Spiraea trilobata Lindl., flowers often white, sepals 5, petals 5, numerous stamens, ovary 5-carpellate, apocarpous, superior.

Rosa multiflora Thunb., flowers pink, sepals 5, petals 5, numerous stamens and carpels, apocarpous, ovary superior.

Prunus persica L., flowers peach, sepals 5, petals 5, numerous stamens, ovary 1-carpellate, with single locules containing 2 ovules, superior.

Chaenomeles spinosa Nakai., flowers pink, sepals 5, petals 5, numerous stamens, ovary 5-carpellate, inferior, syncarpous, 5-loculi with each locules containing numerous ovules.

Which subfamily does the above four plants belong to respectively?

5. Experiment Guides

5.1 Lahoratory Assignments

5.1.1　Write down the flower formula of *Rumex dentatus*., and draw out its flower diagram.

5.1.2　Wrile down the flower formula of *Brassica chinensis*., and draw out its flower diagram.

5.1.3　Write out the flower formula of *Spiraea trilobata* Lindl., *Rosa multiflora* Thunb., *Prunus persica* L., *Chaenomeles spinosa* Nakai., and draw out the flower diagram of *Rosa*

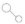

multiflora Thunb. and *Chaenomeles spinosa* Nakai respeccively.

5.1.4　Making use of the subfamily key to retrieval plants of Rosaceae and their subfamilies.

5.2　Questions

5.2.1　Which characters of *Rumex dentatus* represent the characters of Polygonaceae?

5.2.2　What characters do Brassicaceae possess?

5.2.3　What are the differences among the four subfamilies in Rosaceae?

5.2.4　Try to retrieval one unknown plant making use of key.

实验十三 豆科 Leguminosae、伞形科 Umbelliferae、唇形科 Labiatae

一、实验目的

1. 掌握豆科、伞形科、唇形科植物花部的主要特征。
2. 认识一定数量的各科代表药用植物。

二、实验材料

合欢、紫荆、槐、野胡萝卜、益母草。

三、仪器与试剂

显微镜、放大镜、载玻片、镊子、刀片、解剖针、培养皿、擦镜纸。

四、实验步骤

(一) 豆科

仔细观察合欢、紫荆、槐，注意它们花的对称情况、花瓣的卷叠方式、雄蕊的数量和类型（图 2-13-1、图 2-13-2、图 2-13-3）。

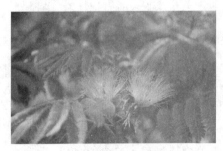

图 13-1 合欢

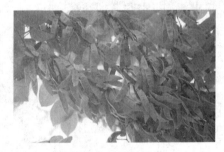

图 13-2 紫荆果实

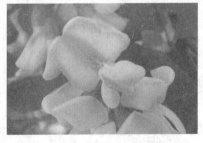

图 13-3 槐花

（二）伞形科

取野胡萝卜的花序观察，其为复伞形花序。取其中的一个伞形花序，认知伞形花序。取花序中一朵花，解剖观察，可见花基数为 5，子房下位，2 心皮合生，2 室，每室胚珠 1。花柱 2，基部膨大成盘状（图 2-13-4）。

（三）唇形科

取益母草，观察其轮伞花序。取其中一朵花，解剖观察，可见花萼钟形，5 裂，花冠二唇形，雄蕊为二强雄蕊，子房上位，2 心皮合生，4 个子房室（图 2-13-5）。

另腊叶标本观察，尽可能地多认识各个科的代表药用植物。

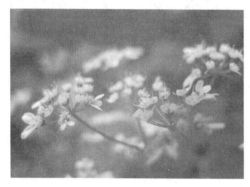
图 2-13-4　野胡萝卜花

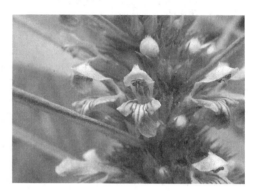
图 2-11-5　益母草轮伞花序

五、实验指导

（一）实验作业

分别写出紫荆、益母草的花程式。

（二）思考题

豆科三亚科有何区别？

Experiment 13　Leguminosae, Umbelliferae, Labiatae

1. Objective

1.1　Master the primary characters of plant flower in Leguminosae, Umbelliferae, Labiatae respectively.

1.2　Understand certain amount of representative medicinal plants in each family.

2. Experiment Materials

Albizia julibrissin Durazz, *Cercis chinensis* Bunge, *Sophora japonica* L., *Daucus carota* L., *Leonurus japonicus* Houtt.

3. Apparatus and Reagents

Microscope, magnifying glass, glass slide, cover glass, dissecting needle, foreceps, blade, culture dish, lens paper.

4. Procedures

4.1　Leguminosae

Carefully anatomize and observe the three provided materials: *Albizia julibrissin* Durazz, *Cercis chinensis* Bunge, *Sophore japonica* L.respectively, while paying special attention to the following questions: symmetrical manner of flowers, fashion of aestivation, amount and type of stamens.

4.2　Umbelliferae

Examine the inflorescence of *Daucus carota* L., found it is the compound umbel, and take up one of umbel (do not pick up flower from the margin of inflorescence, for which is usually a decorating one) for observation under the anatomical lens.

There can be seen that sepals 5, petals 5, often separated, stamens 5, ovary inferior, 2-carpellate, syncarpous, bilocular with single ovule each; style 2, with the base inflated into a discal or flat orbicular shaped stylopodium.

4.3　Labiatae

Pick up *Leonurus japonicus* Houtt, and examine its verticillaster. Dissect the flower under the anatomical lens, note as follows: sepal present in shape of bell, 5-lobed; corolla 2-lipped, division absent in the upper lip, the lower lip 3-lobed, with the mid-lobe obcordate; stamens 4, didynamous stamens, adnate to corolla, ovary superior, 2-carpellate, syncarpous, with 4 locule.

Examine herbarium sheets carefully; understand some amount of representative medicinal plants in each family.

5. Experiment Guides

5.1　Laboratory Assignments

Write out the flower formula of *Cercis chinensis* Bunge and *Leonurus japonicus* Houtt.

5.2　Questions

What are the differences among the three subfamilies Fabaceae?

实验十四　菊科 Asteraceae（Compositae）、禾本科 Poaceae（Gramineae）、百合科 Liliaceae

一、实验目的

1. 掌握各科植物花部的主要特征。
2. 识别一定数量的各科代表药用植物。
3. 能熟练使用检索表，检索未知植物到科、属。

二、实验材料

野菊、小麦、浙贝母。

三、仪器与试剂

显微镜、放大镜、载玻片、镊子、刀片、解剖针、培养皿、擦镜纸。

四、实验步骤

（一）菊科

观察野菊的花序。舌状花黄色，为雌性，花冠不裂，柱头 2 裂，注意观察萼片。管状花两性，纵切开花冠筒，可见有 5 个雄蕊，且为聚药雄蕊；柱头 2 裂，子房下位，1 室，1 胚珠。注意观察管状花有无萼片。（图 2-14-1）

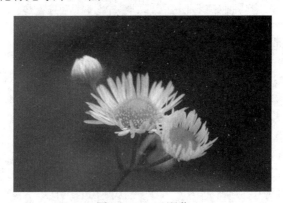

图 2-14-1　野菊

（二）禾本科

观察小麦植物。麦秆具有明显的节和节间；叶由叶鞘、叶片、叶舌、叶耳组成，注意观察叶舌、叶耳的位置。根为须根系。

认识麦穗，即复穗状花序，它是由许多小穗，即穗状花序构成。小穗由 3～5 朵小花组成。小穗下具外颖、内颖，每一小花外有外稃、内稃，外稃硬质，顶端有芒，内稃膜质，两边内卷，浆片 2，很小；雄蕊 3，花药丁字着生；雌蕊 1，柱头 2，羽毛状，子房上位，2～3 心皮合生，1 室，1 胚珠。颖果。（图 2-14-2）

（三）百合科

取浙贝母的花解剖。为典型的三出数五轮花，花被片 6，2 轮，雄蕊 6，2 轮；子房上位，3 心皮合生，3 室，中轴胎座，胚珠多数。注意观察花萼、花瓣是否有区分。（图 2-14-3）

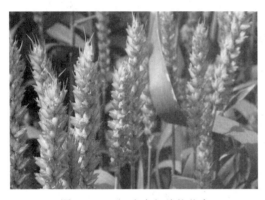
图 2-14-2　小麦复穗状花序

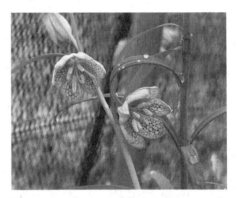
图 2-14-3　浙贝母花

五、实验指导

（一）实验作业

1. 写出野菊的花程式，并绘出其舌状花、管状花的纵剖面图。

2. 写出小麦花的花程式，并绘出小穗结构简图。

3. 写出浙贝母花程式，并绘出花图式。

（二）思考题

1. 禾本科和莎草科有何异同？

2. 百合科的特征是什么？

3. 菊科有何特征？舌状花亚科和管状花亚科有何区别？

Experiment 14　Asteraceae (Compositae), Poaceae (Gramineae), Liliaceae

1. Objective

1.1　Master the floral main characters of plant in each family.

1.2　Recognize certain quantity of representative medical plants in each family.

1.3　Be capable of adroit utilizing identification key in doing survey for unknown plants to their families and genus respective.

2. Experiment Materials

Dendranthema indicus L., *Triticun aestivum* L., *Fritillaria thunbergii* Miq.

3. Apparatus and Reagents

Microscope, magnifying glass, glass slide, cover glass, dissecting needle, forceps, blade, culture dish, lens paper.

4. Procedures

4.1　Asteraceae (Compositae)

Observe the inflorescences of *Dendranthema indicus* L. and not the following tubulous type, the former often yellow, pistillate flowers, corolla untied, stigma 5-lobed, notoce if or not there is any sepal? Tubulous flowers bisexual, and cut the corolla tube longitudinally, there can be seen 5 stamens, which are syngenesious stamens, stigma 5-lobed, ovary inferior, and uniloculate with a single ovule. Note that is there any sepal?

4.2　Poaceae

Examine the plant of *Triticum aestivum* L., found that wheat straw possesses evident nodes and internodes; and the leaf composed of leaf sheath, blade, ligulate and auricle. Note where does ligulate and auricle occur? The root is belonging to fibrous root system.

Learn to recognize ear that is the compound spike, consisted of lots of spikelet, which is called the spike. The spikelet, composed of 3~5 flowerets, under of which bearing outer glume and inner glume, and to the external of each floweret exist inferior palea and plalea. The inferior palea is siereoplasm, with aristae on its top end, while the palea is membranaceous with both sides involution. Lodicules 2, usually very small; stamens 3; anther of versatile, pistil 1, stigmata 2, presenting featheriness-shaped; ovary superior, carpels 2~3, syncarpous, with 1 locules containing single ovule; and fruit a caryopsis.

4.3 Liliaceae

Anatomize flower from *Fritillaria thunbergii* Miq., it is visible that the typical trimerous (having flower parts in sets of three) five-whorl flower; perianth of 6 lodicules, with 2 whorls; stamens 6, with 2 whorls; ovary superior, 3-carpellate, syncarpous, with 3 loculi; axile placenta and numerous ovules. Whether or not there is distinction between sepal and petal?

5. Experiment Guides

5.1 Laboratory Assignments

5.1.1 Write out the flower formula of *Dendranthema indicus* L., and draw out its longitudinal profile chart of ligulate and tubulous flowers.

5.1.2 Write down the flower formula of *Triticum aestivum* L., and sketch the structure of spikelet.

5.1.3 Draw up the flower formula of *Fritillaria thunbergii* Miq., and draw its flower diagram.

5.2 Questions

5.2.1 Depict the similarities and the dissimilarities between Poaceae and Cyperaceae.

5.2.2 What are the characters of Liliaceae?

5.2.3 What are the characters of Asteraceae? And what is the distinction between Liguliglorae and Tubuliflorae?

实验十五　毛茛科 Ranunculaceae、木犀科 Oleaceae、天南星科 Araceae

一、实验目的

1. 掌握毛茛科、木犀科、天南星科植物的主要特征，并认识这几科中的部分药用植物。
2. 初步学会从形态方面鉴别药用植物的方法。

二、仪器用品、实验材料

新鲜材料：小叶女贞。
腊叶标本：乌头、芍药、白头翁、毛茛、天南星、半夏、连翘、女贞。

三、仪器与试剂

解剖镜、解剖针、镊子、培养皿、蒸馏水、吸水纸。

四、实验步骤

（一）毛茛科

取乌头、芍药、白头翁、毛茛等植物的腊叶标本，观察茎、叶、花、果实等方面的特征（图 2-15-1、图 2-15-2），注意叶子是否分裂，雄蕊和心皮是否多数？果实的类型是什么？总结出毛茛科植物的主要特征。

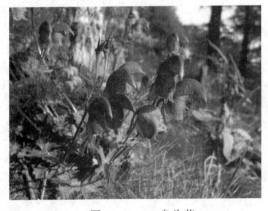

图 2-15-1　乌头花

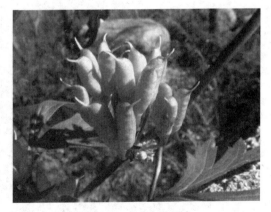

图 2-15-2　乌头果实

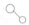

（二）天南星科

观察天南星及半夏的腊叶标本，均有生于地下的块茎，注意两种植物的叶有何不同。花单性，肉穗花序，天南星为雌雄异株，半夏为雌雄同株，雄花生于上部，雌花在下。果实均为浆果。

（三）木犀科

取小叶女贞的新鲜材料，注意叶子的着生方式、花被片的数目和雄蕊的数目。

观察连翘、女贞的腊叶标本，注意茎、叶、花、果实等方面的特征，总结出木犀科植物的主要特征。

五、实验指导

（一）实验作业

1. 绘制小叶女贞花的解剖图，并注明各部分名称。

2. 绘制乌头花的解剖图，并标明各部分名称。

（二）思考题

毛茛科植物的原始性表现在哪些方面？

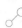

Experiment 15　Ranunculaceae, Oleaceae, Araceae

1. Objective

1.1　Master the main characteristics of Ranunculaceae, Oleaceae, and Araceae, and recognize some of the medicinal plants in these families.

1.2　Preliminary learning to identify medicinal plants in terms of morphology.

2. Experiment Materials

Fresh materials: *Ligustrum quihoui* Carr.

Specimens: *Aconitum carmichaeli* Debx., *Paeonia lactiflora* Pall, *Pulsatilla chinensis* (Bunge) Regel, *Ranunculus japonicus* Thunb., *Arisaema heterophyllum* Blume, *Pinellia ternata* (Thunb.) Breit, *Forsythia suspensa* (Thunb.) Vahl, *Ligustrum lucidum* Ait.

3. Apparatus and Reagents

Microscope, magnifying glass, glass slide, cover glass, dissecting needle, foreceps, blade, culture dish, lens paper.

4. Procedures

4.1　Ranunculaceae

Take the herbarium specimens of *Aconitum carmichaeli*, *Paeonia lactiflora* and *Pycnonotus sinensis*, then observe the characteristics of stem, leaf, flower, fruit and etc., pay attention to whether the leaves are split, and whether the stamens and carpels are multiple? What is the type of fruit? Finally, the main characteristics of Ranunculaceae need to be summarized.

4.2　Araceae

Observe the specimens of *Arisaema heterophyllum* and *Pinellia ternata*. Both of them have underground tubers, pay attention to the differences of two kinds of plant leaves. Please make sure the following conclusions are correct: both are unisexual flower, spadix, *Arisaema heterophyllum* is dioecism, *Pinellia ternata* is monoecism, staminate flower is born at upper, pistillate flower is born below. The type of fruit is berry.

4.3　Oleaceae

Take the fresh material of *Ligustrum quihoui*, notice the arranged pattern of the leaves and the number of tepals and stamens.

When observe the specimens of *Forsythia suspense* and *Ligustrum lucidum*, notice the characteristics of stem, leaf, flower and fruit, and then the main characteristics of the

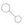

Oleaceaeplant need to be summarized.

5. Experiment Guides

5.1 Laboratory Assignments

5.1.1 Draw the detailed anatomic diagram of *Ligustrum quihoui* flower and indicate the name of each part.

5.1.2 Draw the detailed anatomic diagram of *Aconitum carmichaeli* flower and indicate the name of each part.

5.2 Questions

Why do you think that plants of Ranunculaceae are primitive?

实验十六 植物分类学综合实验

一、实验目的

通过本实验，让学生应用已学过的植物分类学知识，观察植物，解剖植物的花部特征，并通过查找文献及使用检索表来鉴定植物。同时，学会初步的植物资源野外调查工作。

二、实验材料

校园及附近植物。

三、实验步骤

每个同学在校园中任选 10 种植物，仔细观察、记录、解剖。并查阅参考书及检索表来鉴定植物，最好能检索到属甚至种。

利用课余时间进行野外药用植物资源调查，如日照地区唇形科药用植物的调查，校园菊科药用植物的调查等等，这项工作可以多人一组。

四、实验指导

（一）实验作业

1. 写出 10 种植物的检索路线及名称。

2. 写出你的专项野外药用植物资源调查的调查报告。

（二）思考题

1. 学习植物分类学对你的专业有何帮助？

2. 你能讲述出几种现代植物分类学的实验方法？

Experiment 16   Comprehensive Experiment of Plant Taxonomy

1. Objective

Through this experiment, to have students applying the knowledge of plant taxonomy to study plant, to grasp the floral characters by anatomy, and to identify plant using literature retrieval and identification key, on the meanwhile, to make them master the method for field investigation of plant resource.

2. Experiment Materials

Plants in or around the campus.

3. Experiment Content

Every studet chooses ten plants at random in the campus, and make careful observation, note and anatomy. Forever more, you should identify plants using literature retrieval and identification key, and you may as well search out their genus or even species respectively.

And after school, you may do field investigation for resources of medical plants. For example, survey for Labiatae medical plants in the region of Rizhao, or compositae medical plants in the campus and the like. You can do such work in groups.

4. Experiment Guides

4.1   Laboratory Assignments

4.1.1   Write out retrieval ways for 10 plants and their names.

4.1.2   Write out your special field investigation report for the resource of medical plants.

4.2   Questions

4.2.1   In what way to help you in your major by learning the plant taxonomy?

4.2.2   How many expenment methods, could you describe, that applied in the modern plant taxonomy?

实验十七　CTAB 法提取植物基因组 DNA

一、实验目的

学习从植物组织中（幼叶）提取基因组 DNA 的基本原理和方法。

二、实验原理

采用机械研磨的方法破碎植物的组织和细胞，在液氮中研磨，材料易于破碎。CTAB（十六烷基三甲基溴化铵），是一种阳离子去污剂，可溶解细胞膜并与核酸形成复合物。该复合物在高盐的溶液中（＞0.7 mol/L NaCl）是可溶的，通过有机溶剂抽提，去除蛋白、多糖、酚类等杂质后加入乙醇或异丙醇沉淀（CTAB 能溶于乙醇或异丙醇）即可使核酸分离出来。

三、实验材料

新鲜的植物叶片。

四、仪器与试剂

抽提液［如 100 ml 抽提液的配制：2% CTAB 2 g，1 mol/L Tris（pH 8.0）10 ml，0.5 mol/L EDTA（pH 8.0）4 ml，5 mol/L NaCl 28 ml，最后加双蒸水定容至 100 ml］，三氯甲烷/异戊醇（24:1），异丙醇，70%乙醇，液氮。研钵、微量移液器、枪头、EP 管、高速离心机、恒温水浴摇床。

五、实验步骤

1. 取幼嫩的植物叶片剪碎，倒入液氮迅速研磨成粉，转入 1.5 ml 离心管内。加入等体积的 65 ℃预热的 DNA 提取缓冲液（约 500 μl），置于 65 ℃的恒温水浴摇床上 30 分钟～1 小时。

2. 加入等体积的三氯甲烷:异戊醇（24:1）（约 500 μl），轻轻上下颠倒 5 分钟，静置 5 分钟，之后于 12000 rpm 离心 10 分钟。

3. 吸取上层水相，重复步骤 2 一次。

4. 吸取上层水相，加入预冷 2/3 体积的异丙醇，轻缓颠倒 2 分钟并置－20 ℃冰箱内 30 分钟。

5. 待 DNA 沉淀后于 12000 rpm 离心收集，收集的 DNA 于 70%乙醇中洗 2～3 次。将弃去乙醇风干后的 DNA 加适量水使其溶解，－20 ℃保存待用。

六、注意事项

1. 液氮温度为 –196 ℃，研磨时需要戴厚手套，注意安全。

2. 抽取上清液时应把枪头剪掉下端，以防 DNA 破碎。

3. 离心时，应该配平。

七、实验指导

（一）实验作业

结合原理，简述 CTAB 法分离植物总 DNA 的基本过程。

（二）思考题

为了获得高质量的植物总基因组 DNA，在分离提取中应该注意哪些问题？

Experiment 17　Plant genome DNA extraction
by CTAB methods

1. Objective

Learn the basic principles and methods of extracting genomic DNA from plant tissue (young leaves).

2. Experiment Principle

The tissue and cells of the plant were crushed by mechanical grinding, and the materials were easily broken in the liquid nitrogen. CTAB (hexadecyl trimethyl ammonium bromide) was a cationic detergent which can dissolve the cell membrane and form a complex with nucleic acid. The compound in high salt solution (> 0.7 mol/L NaCl) is soluble, remove impurities such as protein, polysaccharide by organic solvent extraction, and then added ethanol or isopropanol (CTAB was soluble in ethanol or isopropanol) in order to make nucleic acid precipitate and separate.

3. Experiment Reagents

Young leaves of fresh plant.

4. Experiment instruments

The extraction liquid (Such as 100 ml extraction solution: 2% CTAB 2 g, 1 mol/L Tris (pH 8.0) 10 ml, 0.5 mol/L EDTA (pH 8.0) 4 ml, 5 mol/L NaCl 28 ml, and then add double distilled water to 100 ml), chloroform/isoamyl alcohol (24:1), isopropanol, 70% alcohol, liquid nitrogen. Mortar, micropipette, pipette head, EP tube, high speed centrifuge, thermostatic water bath.

5. Experiment Contents

5.1　Young plant leaves are shredded and grinded into powder in the liquid nitrogen, then they are poured into a 1.5 ml centrifuge tube. Add the equal volume 65 ℃ preheated DNA extraction liquid (500 μl) into this centrifuge tube, and then place this centrifuge tube on a constant temperature shaking bath at 65 ℃ for 30 min~1 h.

5.2　Add equal volume of chloroform/iso-amyl alcohol (24:1) (500 μl), mix for about 5 min. Let sit for five minutes, then spin at 12,000 rpm for 10 min.

5.3　Absorb the upper water phase and repeat step 2 once.

5.4　Absorb the upper water phase, add cold 2/3 volume of isopropanol. Then place it in refrigerator at −20 ℃ for 30 minutes after reversing gently for 2 minutes.

5.5　Spin at 12,000 rpm in order to collect DNA precipitation. Collected DNA precipitation was washed 2～3 times in 70% ethanol. Dissolve the air-dried DNA with proper amount of water and preserve at −20 ℃.

6. Notice

6.1　The liquid nitrogen temperature is −196 ℃, grind carefully with thick gloves when grinding.

6.2　Cut off the end of the muzzle to prevent the DNA from breaking.

6.3　When centrifuging, it should be balanced.

7. Experiment Guides

7.1　Laboratory Assignments

Based on the principle, the basic process of plants total DNA extraction using CTAB method was introduced.

7.2　Questions

In order to obtain high quality plant total genomic DNA, what should be paid attention to in separating extraction?